Advanced and Metastatic Renal Cell Carcinoma

Editors

WILLIAM C. HUANG
EZEQUIEL BECHER

UROLOGIC CLINICS
OF NORTH AMERICA

www.urologic.theclinics.com

Consulting Editor
SAMIR S. TANEJA

August 2020 • Volume 47 • Number 3

ELSEVIER

1600 John F. Kennedy Boulevard • Suite 1800 • Philadelphia, Pennsylvania, 19103-2899

http://www.theclinics.com

UROLOGIC CLINICS OF NORTH AMERICA Volume 47, Number 3
August 2020 ISSN 0094-0143, ISBN-13: 978-0-323-75541-2

Editor: Kerry Holland
Developmental Editor: Julia McKenzie

Urologic Clinics of North America (ISSN 0094-0143) is published quarterly by Elsevier Inc., 360 Park Avenue South, New York, NY 10010-1710. Months of issue are February, May, August, and November. Business and Editorial Offices: 1600 John F. Kennedy Blvd., Suite 1800, Philadelphia, PA 19103-2899. Periodicals postage paid at New York, NY and additional mailing offices. Subscription prices are $391.00 per year (US individuals), $795.00 per year (US institutions), $100.00 per year (US students and residents), $450.00 per year (Canadian individuals), $993.00 per year (Canadian institutions), $100.00 per year (Canadian students/residents), $520.00 per year (foreign individuals), $993.00 per year (foreign institutions), and $240.00 per year (foreign students/residents). Foreign air speed delivery is included in all *Clinics* subscription prices. All prices are subject to change without notice. **POSTMASTER:** Send address changes to *Urologic Clinics of North America*, Elsevier Health Sciences Division, Subscription Customer Service, 3251 Riverport Lane, Maryland Heights, MO 63043. **Customer Service: 1-800-654-2452 (US). From outside the United States, call 1-314-447-8871. Fax: 1-314-447-8029. E-mail: JournalsCustomerServiceusa@elsevier.com (for print support)** and **JournalsOnlineSupport-usa@elsevier.com (for online support)**.

Reprints. For copies of 100 or more, of articles in this publication, please contact the Commercial Reprints Department, Elsevier Inc., 360 Park Avenue South, New York, New York 10010-1710. Tel.: 212-633-3874; Fax: 212-633-3820; E-mail: reprints@elsevier.com.

Urologic Clinics of North America is covered in MEDLINE/PubMed (*Index Medicus*), *Excerpta Medica, Current Contents/Clinical Medicine, Science Citation Index,* and *ISI/BIOMED.*

Contributors

CONSULTING EDITOR

SAMIR S. TANEJA, MD
The James M. Neissa and Janet Riha Neissa
Professor of Urologic Oncology, Professor of
Urology, Radiology, and Biomedical
Engineering, GU Program Leader, Perlmutter
Cancer Center, Director, Division of Urologic
Oncology, Department of Urology, NYU
Langone Health, New York, New York, USA

EDITORS

WILLIAM C. HUANG, MD, FACS
Associate Professor of Urologic Oncology,
NYU Grossman School of Medicine, Chief of
Urology, Tisch Hospital, Co-Director, NYU
Langone Robotic Surgery Center, NYU
Langone Health, Perlmutter Cancer Center,
New York, New York, USA

EZEQUIEL BECHER, MD
Urologic Oncology Fellow, Department of
Urology, NYU Langone Health, New York, New
York, USA

AUTHORS

EDWIN JASON ABEL, MD, FACS
Associate Professor, Department of Urology,
University of Wisconsin-Madison School of
Medicine and Public Health, Madison,
Wisconsin, USA

MOHAMAD E. ALLAF, MD
Vice Chairman and Professor of Urology,
Oncology, and Biomedical Engineering,
Director of Minimally Invasive and Robotic
Surgery, Department of Urology, Brady
Urological Institute, Johns Hopkins School of
Medicine, Baltimore, Maryland, USA

ZEYNEP E. ARSLAN, MD
Istanbul Medipol University Medical School,
Istanbul, Turkey

KYROLLIS ATTALLA, MD
Department of Surgery, Urology Service,
Memorial Sloan Kettering Cancer Center, New
York, New York, USA

EZEQUIEL BECHER, MD
Urologic Oncology Fellow, Department of
Urology, NYU Langone Health, New York, New
York, USA

MICHAEL J. BILES, MD
Department of Urology, The James Buchanan
Brady Urological Institute, Johns Hopkins
School of Medicine, Baltimore, Maryland,
USA

VIJAY DAMARLA, MD
Decatur Memorial Hospital, Decatur, Illinois,
USA

NAZLI DIZMAN, MD
Department of Medical Oncology and
Experimental Therapeutics, City of Hope
Comprehensive Cancer Center, Duarte,
California, USA

NICHOLAS DONIN, MD
Assistant Clinical Professor, Division of
Urologic Oncology, Department of Urology,
David Geffen School of Medicine at UCLA, Los
Angeles, California, USA

MATTHEW FENG
Department of Medical Oncology and
Experimental Therapeutics, City of Hope
Comprehensive Cancer Center, Duarte,
California, USA

RONAN FLIPPOT, MD
Dana-Farber Cancer Institute, Lank Center for
Genitourinary Oncology, Boston,
Massachusetts, USA; Department of Cancer
Medicine, Gustave Roussy, Villejuif, France

BORIS GERSHMAN, MD
Division of Urologic Surgery, Beth Israel
Deaconess Medical Center, Boston,
Massachusetts, USA

GEORGE GOUCHER, BHSc, MD
Urology Resident, Department of Surgery,
Division of Urology, McMaster University,
McMaster Institute of Urology, St. Joseph's
Healthcare Hamilton, Hamilton, Ontario,
Canada

A ARI HAKIMI, MD
Department of Surgery, Urology Service,
Memorial Sloan Kettering Cancer Center, New
York, New York, USA

BRYAN DR HALL, BA
Medical Student, Department of Urology,
University of Wisconsin-Madison School of
Medicine and Public Health, Madison,
Wisconsin, USA

JEN HOOGENES, MS, MSc, PhD
Department of Surgery, Division of Urology,
McMaster University, McMaster Institute of
Urology, St. Joseph's Healthcare Hamilton,
Hamilton, Ontario, Canada

WILLIAM C. HUANG, MD, FACS
Associate Professor of Urologic Oncology,
NYU Grossman School of Medicine, Chief of
Urology, Tisch Hospital, Co-Director, NYU
Langone Robotic Surgery Center, NYU

Langone Health, Perlmutter Cancer Center,
New York, New York, USA

DORA JERICEVIC, MD
Department of Urology, NYU Langone Health,
New York, New York, USA

KIMBERLY L. JOHUNG, MD, PhD
Associate Professor, Therapeutic Radiology,
Yale School of Medicine, Yale Therapeutic
Radiology, New Haven, Connecticut,
USA

SUNG JUN MA, MD
Resident Physician, Department of
Radiation Medicine, Roswell Park
Comprehensive Cancer Center, Buffalo, New
York, USA

STELLA K. KANG, MD, MSc
Departments of Radiology and Population
Health, NYU Langone Medical Center, New
York, New York, USA

ANIL KAPOOR, BSc, BEng, MD, FRCSC
Department of Surgery, Division of Urology,
McMaster University, McMaster Institute of
Urology, St. Joseph's Healthcare Hamilton,
Hamilton, Ontario, Canada

JOSE A. KARAM, MD
Assistant Professor, Department of Urology,
The University of Texas MD Anderson Cancer
Center, Houston, Texas, USA

JAEHOON KIM, BHSc, MD (Candidate)
McMaster University Michael G. Degroote
School of Medicine, Hamilton, Ontario,
Canada

BRADLEY A. McGREGOR, MD
Dana-Farber Cancer Institute, Lank Center for
Genitourinary Oncology, Boston,
Massachusetts, USA

JOSEPH A. MICCIO, MD
Resident Physician, Department of
Therapeutic Radiology, Yale School of
Medicine, New Haven, Connecticut, USA

OLUWADAMILOLA T. OLADERU, MD
Resident Physician, Harvard Radiation
Oncology Program, Massachusetts General
Hospital, Boston, Massachusetts, USA

ARIA F. OLUMI, MD
Division of Urologic Surgery, Beth Israel
Deaconess Medical Center, Boston,
Massachusetts, USA

SUMANTA K. PAL, MD
Department of Medical Oncology and
Experimental Therapeutics, City of Hope
Comprehensive Cancer Center, Duarte,
California, USA

HITEN D. PATEL, MD, MPH
Department of Urology, The James Buchanan
Brady Urological Institute, Johns Hopkins
School of Medicine, Baltimore, Maryland, USA

DANIEL D. SHAPIRO, MD
Department of Urology, The University of
Texas MD Anderson Cancer Center, Houston,
Texas, USA

BRIAN SHUCH, MD
Associate Professor of Urology, Director,
Kidney Cancer Program, Division of Urologic
Oncology, Department of Urology, David
Geffen School of Medicine at UCLA, Los
Angeles, California, USA

POOJA UNADKAT, MD
Division of Urologic Surgery, Beth Israel
Deaconess Medical Center, Boston,
Massachusetts, USA

SOUMYA V.L. VIG, MD
Department of Radiology, NYU Langone
Medical Center, New York, New York, USA

MARTIN H. VOSS, MD
Department of Medicine, Memorial Sloan
Kettering Cancer Center, New York, New York,
USA

STANLEY WENG, MS
Department of Surgery, Urology Service,
Memorial Sloan Kettering Cancer Center, New
York, New York, USA

MARY E. WESTERMAN, MD
Department of Urology, The University Texas
MD Anderson Cancer Center, Houston, Texas,
USA

CHRISTOPHER G. WOOD, MD
Professor, Department of Urology, The
University of Texas MD Anderson Cancer
Center, Houston, Texas, USA

ERIKA WOOD, MD, MPH
Resident Physician, Department of Urology,
David Geffen School of Medicine at UCLA, Los
Angeles, California, USA

ELCIN ZAN, MD
Department of Radiology, NYU Langone
Medical Center, New York, New York,
USA

Contents

Advanced renal cell carcinoma is not uncommon, but necessitates a multidisciplinary approach for optimal treatment. Targeted therapy has increased the likelihood of urologists managing patients in all disease stages. Neoadjuvant therapy is currently experimental. Systemic therapy for metastatic disease demonstrates survival benefits. The role of cytoreductive nephrectomy and adjuvant therapy is dependent on patient selection. Management of advanced renal cell carcinoma involves continued optimization of available agents and biomarker development. This article reviews the role of the urologist in medical and surgical therapies, including prognostication, management of locally advanced and metastatic disease, and provides the most recent clinical trial data.

Patients with renal cell carcinoma may develop metastases after radical nephrectomy, and therefore monitoring with imaging for recurrent or metastatic disease is critical. Imaging varies with specific suspected site of disease. Computed tomography/MRI of the abdomen and pelvis are mainstay modalities. Osseous and central nervous system imaging is reserved for symptomatic patients. Radiologic reporting is evolving to reflect effects of systemic therapy on lesion morphology. Nuclear medicine studies compliment routine imaging as newer agents are evaluated for more accurate tumor staging. Imaging research aims to fill gaps in treatment selection and monitoring of treatment response in metastatic renal cell carcinoma.

In the preceding two decades, several milestones have been reached in the management of patients with metastatic renal cell carcinoma (mRCC), including the development of novel targeted agents paralleling an increased understanding of the molecular biology of this disease process. Recently, a renewed enthusiasm for immunotherapy in the form of immune checkpoint blockade has resulted in significant strides in the treatment of mRCC. Despite these advances, treatment remains challenging for clinicians, and only modest survival benefits are observed with current treatment paradigms. The risk-stratification tools and investigated predictive and prognostic biomarkers in patients with mRCC are detailed in this review.

Cytoreductive Nephrectomy in the Era of Tyrosine Kinase and Immuno-Oncology Checkpoint Inhibitors   359

Michael J. Biles, Hiten D. Patel, and Mohamad E. Allaf

The role for cytoreductive nephrectomy (CN) in the treatment of metastatic renal cell carcinoma (mRCC) has evolved with advancements in systemic therapy. During the cytokine-based immunotherapy era, CN provided a clear survival benefit and was considered standard of care in management of mRCC. The development of targeted systemic therapy directed at the vascular endothelial growth factor pathway altered the treatment paradigm and accentuated the importance of risk stratification in treatment selection. This article reviews the literature evaluating the benefit of CN during the evolution of systemic therapy and provides clinical recommendations for current utilization of CN in patients with mRCC.

The Role of Lymphadenectomy in Patients with Advanced Renal Cell Carcinoma   371

Pooja Unadkat, Aria F. Olumi, and Boris Gershman

The role of lymph node dissection (LND) in the management of renal cell carcinoma (RCC) is controversial. LND serves an indisputable staging role by providing pathologic nodal stage. However, while earlier observational studies had suggested a survival benefit to LND, more recent observational evidence and a randomized trial do not support a survival benefit. The majority of patients with isolated lymph node involvement appear to harbor occult metastatic disease. Still, LND is not associated with increased perioperative morbidity when performed in experienced centers. LND may therefore play a predominantly staging role in patients at increased risk of lymph node metastases.

The Evolving Role of Metastasectomy for Patients with Metastatic Renal Cell Carcinoma   379

Bryan DR Hall and Edwin Jason Abel

Surgical metastasectomy continues to be utilized for patients with solitary or low-volume metastatic renal cell carcinoma (mRCC). Although few high-quality data are available to evaluate outcomes, local treatment is recommended when feasible because it may allow a subset of patients to delay or avoid systemic treatments. With the development of improved mRCC therapies, utilization of metastasectomy has increased because most patients have incomplete responses to systemic treatment of their metastases. This review discusses the rationale and history of metastasectomy, trends in utilization, prognostic factors for patient selection, site-specific considerations, alternatives for nonsurgical local treatment, and risk of morbidity associated with metastasectomy.

Minimally Invasive Surgery for Patients with Locally Advanced and/or Metastatic Renal Cell Carcinoma   389

Ezequiel Becher, Dora Jericevic, and William C. Huang

Despite advances in systemic therapy and immunotherapy, surgery continues to have a role in management of advanced renal cell carcinoma (aRCC). Minimally invasive surgery (MIS) is considered standard of care for smaller, localized tumors due to faster recovery without compromising oncologic outcomes. There are concerns about MIS for aRCC due to a potential risk of inferior oncologic outcomes and unusual patterns of disease recurrence. Recent studies, however, suggest that in properly selected patients with aRCC, MIS can provide improved peri-operative outcomes without compromising oncologic control.

Stereotactic radiosurgery and stereotactic body radiation therapy (SBRT) have led to a resurgence of the use of radiotherapy in the management of advanced renal cell carcinoma (RCC). These techniques provide excellent local control and palliation of metastatic sites of disease with minimal toxicity. Additionally, SBRT to the primary tumor may be efficacious and well tolerated in select patients that are not surgical candidates. Emerging data suggest that SBRT may potentiate the immune response, and current and future study will evaluate if SBRT can improve survival outcomes in patients with metastatic RCC.

UROLOGIC CLINICS OF NORTH AMERICA

SERIES OF RELATED INTEREST:
Hematology/Oncology Clinics of North America
http://www.hemonc.theclinics.com/

Preface
Current Landscape of Advanced and Metastatic Renal Cell Carcinoma Management

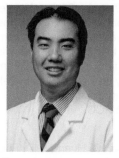
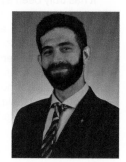

William C. Huang, MD, FACS   Ezequiel Becher, MD

Editors

The first decade of the new millennium witnessed a revolution in the management of advanced renal cell carcinoma (aRCC), thanks to the approval of therapeutic agents targeting the VEGF and mTOR pathways. These targeted therapies transformed the treatment landscape of aRCC and highlighted the success of translational medicine. The arrival of the following decade brought with it clinical trials demonstrating efficacy of immune-oncology (IO) agents in metastatic renal cell carcinoma (mRCC). These trials led to the establishment of second-/third-line roles of IO in mRCC, first as monotherapy and, later, as combinations with other IO agents blocking various immune pathways (ipilimumab/nivolumab). Finally, as the decade came to an end, further successes were achieved through the approval of additional targeted and IO agents and the combination of these therapies resulting in a first line indication across all risk groups with pembolizumab and axitinib (pembrolizumab/axitinib).

All of these treatment advances have resulted in a redefining of the traditional roles of urologists, medical oncologists, and radiation oncologists. Therefore, we have decided to kick-off this issue of *Urologic Clinics* with an article by Kim and colleagues summarizing the evolving role urologist in this new era.

Significant advances have also been made not only on the treatment but also in the evaluation and assessment of patients with aRCC. In the article by Vig and colleagues, the authors examined the evolution of different imaging modalities for diagnosis and staging of aRCC and provide insight on new imaging modalities currently under development.

With the approval of new therapies comes a revision of risk stratification, treatment indications, and patient selection. In the article written by Atalla and colleagues, the authors review the current methods of risk stratification utilizing clinical parameters and discuss the future development of biomarkers that will help identify patients most likely to benefit from these novel therapies.

Changes in indications and sequencing of these drugs continue to change at a dizzying pace. The article by Dizman and colleagues helps clear the confusion by explaining the fundamentals of these agents, providing easy-to-use algorithms, and discussing how gene expression models may play in the near future.

urologic.theclinics.com

Urol Clin N Am 47 (2020) xiii–xiv
https://doi.org/10.1016/j.ucl.2020.05.001
0094-0143/20/© 2020 Published by Elsevier Inc.

There remain, of course, many unanswered questions in this new landscape. Some of these questions revolve around the utilization of these new therapies in patients with non–clear cell histology and how these therapies can be incorporated into use in the perioperative setting. Filppot and colleagues discuss the successes and shortcomings of treating patients with non–clear cell aRCC in their article. Westerman and colleagues elaborate on both completed and ongoing clinical trials in the neoadjuvant setting in their article, while Wood and colleagues discuss the current role of adjuvant therapy and also explore ongoing clinical trials on this subject.

Thanks to the success of these novel therapies, the role of surgery in aRCC continues to be redefined. Biles and colleagues tackle the increasingly controvertial question of cytoreductive nephrectomy in lieu of the seminal findings noted in the CARMENA and SURTIME trials. The benefits of lymphadenectomy and metastasectomy in this era are elegantly discussed and assessed by Unadkat and colleagues and Hall and colleagues, respectively. The articles discussing surgery in aRCC are concluded in a chapter by Becher and colleagues discussing the role of minimally invasive surgery and how the wide acceptance of robotic platforms in the urologic community has impacted the surgical treatment of this disease.

Although much of the focus in advances in the treatment of aRCC revolves around systemic and surgical therapies, other treatment options have continued to evolve as well. RCC has classically been categorized as a radioresistant tumor. However, the advent of higher dose-per-fraction systems has enabled investigators to reevaluate the role of radiotherapy in both localized and mRCC. Miccio and colleagues elaborate on the growing body of evidence behind the rationale for the use of radiation as a beneficial treatment modality in advanced and metastatic RCC.

It has truly been a privilege for us to be guest editors of this issue of *Urologic Clinics*. We feel indebted to all the authors who contributed their knowledge and wisdom as they are the preeminent thought-leaders in this field. It is our wish that this issue will serve in this unprecented time as a road map for not ony urologists, but all health care providers tasked with treating patients with advanced and metastatic RCC.

William C. Huang, MD, FACS
Department of Urology
NYU Langone Health
222 East 41st, 12th Floor
New York, NY 10017, USA

Ezequiel Becher, MD
Department of Urology
NYU Langone Health
222 East 41st, 12th Floor
New York, NY 10017, USA

E-mail addresses:
William.huang@nyulangone.org (W.C. Huang)
Ezequiel.becher@nyulangone.org (E. Becher)

Evolving Role of Urologists in the Management of Advanced Renal Cell Carcinoma

Anil Kapoor, BSc, BEng, MD, FRCSC*, Jaehoon Kim, BHSc, MD (Candidate),
George Goucher, BHSc, MD, Jen Hoogenes, MS, MSc, PhD

KEYWORDS

- Advanced renal cell carcinoma • Metastatic renal cell carcinoma adjuvant therapy
- Neoadjuvant therapy • Cytoreductive nephrectomy • Immune checkpoint inhibitors
- Targeted therapy

KEY POINTS

- Advanced renal cell carcinoma needs proper prognostication to develop an appropriate strategy for surgical and/or medical management.
- Neoadjuvant therapy with tyrosine kinase inhibitors is not well-established, but is a promising avenue for advanced locoregional renal cell carcinoma.
- Immune checkpoint inhibitors show survival benefits in metastatic renal cell carcinoma across stratification groups.
- Cytoreductive nephrectomy and adjuvant therapy should highlight the importance of patient selection.
- Urologists are more likely to manage patients in all stages of renal cell carcinoma owing to the development of systemic therapies.

INTRODUCTION

Kidney cancer accounts for 2.2% of global incidence of cancer, with approximately 400,000 patients and 175,000 deaths annually.[1] The highest estimated incidence for kidney cancer is in North America, with the most common form being renal cell carcinoma (RCC), which accounts for 90% of all primary kidney neoplasms.[2] Owing to the increasing use of abdominal and pelvic imaging, most RCCs are detected incidentally. RCC is usually asymptomatic and more than 17% of patients have distant metastases at clinical presentation that are not amenable to curative surgical resection.[3]

The management of RCC depends on grading and staging through histologic subtypes and tumor extent, with urologists performing surgical resection for earlier disease. Advanced RCCs, which include tumors in pT3-4 of the TNM classification and/or extrarenal involvement (nodal and metastatic), often require a multimodal approach to treatment by incorporating both medical and surgical treatments. The systemic nature of advanced RCC allows urologists to work in a multidisciplinary setting in collaboration with medical and radiation oncologists, palliative care physicians, and other surgical specialties. Urologists have traditionally been responsible for the surgical arm of management for curative, cytoreductive, and palliative purposes. Typically, urologists are the first point of contact at RCC diagnosis and are therefore in a unique position to provide

Division of Urology, Department of Surgery, McMaster University, McMaster Institute of Urology, St. Joseph's Healthcare Hamilton, 50 Charlton Avenue East, Room G334, Hamilton, Ontario L8N 4A6, Canada
* Corresponding author.
E-mail address: akapoor@mcmaster.ca

Urol Clin N Am 47 (2020) 271–280
https://doi.org/10.1016/j.ucl.2020.04.006
0094-0143/20/© 2020 Elsevier Inc. All rights reserved.

guidance throughout the course of a patient's disease management.

Historically, the role of medical therapy with RCC was largely reserved for medical oncologists familiar with common cytotoxic agents and their potential adverse effects. The contemporary role of urologists has shifted to manage patients in all stages of kidney cancer, to provide systemic therapy in addition to surgical care. The advent of targeted therapies, such as tyrosine kinase inhibitors (TKIs) and immune checkpoint inhibitors (ICIs), have increased the arsenal against advanced RCC, with urologists and medical oncologists sharing the role in administering these agents. Moreover, the increased indications for systemic agents for other urologic malignancies, such as ICIs for metastatic urothelial cancers, prompt urologists to accommodate these therapeutic options in their practice.[4] This article explores the emerging role of urologists in the management of locally advanced and metastatic RCC, with an emphasis on contemporary advances in medical therapy and surgical practices.

PROGNOSTICATION
Prognostic and Risk Stratification Tools

Early diagnosis and risk stratification is vital in the management of RCC to provide the appropriate level of care for patients in advanced stages of disease. The early recognition of disease progression can guide the urologist in patient care and treatment decision making, which includes determining whether to approach treatment in a predominantly surgical sense, or to adopt a medical approach, which is one that is currently emerging in this field. Several risk factors in prognostication are outlined in **Table 1**.

In terms of prognosis for advanced locoregional RCC, increased tumor size in pT3a disease has been associated with decreased 10-year survival rates (77%, 54%, and 46% for <4 cm, 4–7 cm, and >7 cm, respectively), and increased tumor and nodal grade through TNM classification is associated with poorer prognosis.[5,6] Postoperative tools and nomograms (eg, Leibovich; UCLA Integrated Staging System; Kattan) are available based on histopathologic features, but are not routinely used in clinical practice.[7]

The prognosis for metastatic disease is largely assessed using the International Metastatic RCC Database Consortium risk score, which incorporates risk factors that include less than 1 year from diagnosis to treatment, Karnofsky performance status of less than 80%, anemia, thrombocytosis, hypercalcemia, and neutrophilia.[8] This externally validated tool stratifies patients into favorable-, intermediate-, and poor-risk groups. The development of molecular markers in tumor pathology will further enhance the ability to stratify patients into risk groups.[7]

Preoperative Biopsy

A percutaneous renal biopsy (PRB) provides important diagnostic information in the presence of incidental small renal masses (≤4 cm), but is not routinely recommended for locally advanced RCC outside of a clinical trial. In cases of metastatic or suspected metastatic disease, renal mass biopsy, or biopsy of a metastatic lesion is recommended to confirm diagnosis.[9] PRBs are not generally indicated for surgical candidates with advanced RCC, because it will not alter the treatment course and the resected sample is superior to cores from PRB.

PRB can identify histologic features for prognosis and guiding of systemic therapies, and often this will be required by a medical oncologist before the initiation of any systemic therapy.[10] Alarming histologic features, such as sarcomatoid differentiation and high Fuhrman nuclear grade (III–IV), suggest poor prognosis and aggressive disease. First-line treatment options are also less effective with non–clear cell subtypes (eg, papillary, chromophobe), because recommendations used from clinical trials largely constitute the clear cell subtype population.[11,12] Currently, the 2019 Canadian guideline recommends newer combination therapies (ipilimumab plus nivolumab, and axitinib plus pembrolizumab) for non–clear cell subtypes based on subgroup analyses of recent adjuvant therapy trials.[13] The lack of conclusive prospective clinical trials for non–clear cell subtypes predispose urologists to manage these patients on an individualized basis and by enrollment into available clinical trials. Molecular profiling of biopsy samples (eg, programmed cell death 1 [PD-1] and PD ligand 1 [PD-L1] for clear cell RCC, MET for type 1 papillary RCC) identifies potential future targets of therapy.[14] Currently, molecular profiling is performed for clinical trials, because most targeted therapies against molecular markers in non–clear cell subtypes are experimental (eg, MET inhibitors for papillary RCC) and the immunotherapy effects on clear cell subtypes expressing PD-1/PD-L1 are still under investigation.[15]

Furthermore, the diagnostic value of PRB for advanced RCCs has not been clearly established. A recent meta-analysis of 7 studies suggests that PRBs have a sensitivity of 99.7% (95% confidence interval [CI], 81.5–100) and specificity of 98.2% (95% CI, 83.3–99.8) in detecting renal malignancies. However, PRB was not able to easily

Table 1
Risk factors that affect disease relapse organized into anatomic (TNM classification) histologic, clinical, and molecular factors

Anatomic	Histologic	Clinical	Molecular[a]
High tumor grade	Collecting duct	Eastern Cooperative	Carbonix anhydrase
Tumor size >4 cm	carcinoma	Oncology Group	IX
Extrarenal	Medullary carcinoma	performance	Hypoxia-inducible
involvement of	Elements of	status >0	factor
tumor	sarcomatoid and	Cachexia	PD-L1 expression
Presence of nodal	rhabdoid	Anemia	PTEN
metastasis	dedifferentiation	Thrombocytosis	Bcl-2
		Elevated erythrocyte	E-cadherins
		sedimentation rate	icroRNAs
		Elevated C-reactive	
		protein	

[a] Molecular factor group shows genes that are often mutated that suggest poor prognosis, but are not currently used in a clinical setting.

identify tumor grade owing to intratumoral heterogeneity of advanced tumors.[16] The sensitivity and specificity is likely lower for advanced RCCs owing to sampling bias of PRB studies with a large proportion of lower grade tumors. Although PRB is a relatively safe procedure and commonly used for active surveillance of small renal masses, owing to its superior diagnostic value it is still under investigation for use in advanced disease.

MANAGEMENT OF LOCALLY ADVANCED DISEASE
Neoadjuvant Therapy

Neoadjuvant therapy is preoperative systemic therapy incorporated with curative intent. The reasoning behind neoadjuvant therapy is to decrease tumor burden (ie, size, complexity), to prevent RCC recurrence, and to eradicate micrometastases.[17] Multiple phase II trials have demonstrated primary tumor size reductions through the effects of TKIs including pazopanib, sunitinib, sorafenib, and axitinib on nonmetastatic RCC.[18–23] Sunitinib was explored in 3 different contexts, where trials including metastatic RCC patients demonstrated a mean reduction in tumor size prospectively (21.1% [range, 3.2%–45%] and 11.8% [range, −11% to 27%]) and median reduction retrospectively (18% [interquartile range, 7%–27%]), and showed that neoadjuvant therapy does not necessarily increase perioperative complications.[18,19,21] Other phase II trials found median tumor size decreases through treatment with pazopanib (26%; before vs after pazopanib: 7.3 cm vs 5.5 cm; $P<.0001$), sorafenib (20.5%; before vs after sorafenib: 7.8 cm vs 6.2 cm; $P<.001$), and axitinib (28.3%; range, 5.3%–

42.9%).[20,22,23] Moreover, intraoperative complications were minimal after TKI administration.[24] There is no consensus regarding inferior vena cava thrombi, as 2 retrospective studies demonstrated opposing conclusions for the role of neoadjuvant therapy in downstaging the tumor; thus, the surgical approach for these particular cases are controversial.[22,25] Despite promising results from clinical trials, neoadjuvant therapy remains in the experimental stages because the findings have shown a low level of objective response rate (ORR) and evidence from large prospective placebo-controlled trials is lacking. Currently, it is not recommended to pursue neoadjuvant therapy for locally advanced RCC outside of a clinical trial, but further investigation is underway to guide its use as a future therapeutic option.

Surgical Management

The definitive treatment for localized RCC is surgical resection; however, the approach becomes more complicated in the presence of a locally advanced tumor. The standard approach for RCC is partial or radical nephrectomy, using an open, laparoscopic, or robot-assisted approach. The efficacy of each procedure is similar, but laparoscopic and robot-assisted are both associated with less morbidity, especially in locoregional tumors.[26–28] This section will focus on considerations for lymphadenectomy (LA), adrenalectomy, and thrombectomy in the management of locally advanced tumors.

The current surgical approach for regional lymph node involvement (pN+) is LA, but it has inconclusive survival benefits, especially for locally advanced disease.[29] A phase III trial showed that radical nephrectomy plus LA resulted in similar morbidity and mortality compared with radical nephrectomy alone, but could not demonstrate overall survival (OS) benefits.[30] The same study included tumors of T1-3 and showed low rates of nodal involvement (4%), hence clinically favorable patients likely clouded the lack of survival benefit for high-risk patients. A recent large retrospective analysis (n = 2722) indicated no difference in OS in patients receiving LA after adjusting for cohort differences.[31] Despite statistical adjustments, there is a risk of bias because the LA cohort contained more advanced disease compared with controls, as expected (48% vs 22% with pT3a or higher). Although the role of LA for survival is unanswered, it is currently an important tool for prognosis, and high-risk groups may still benefit after clinical, radiologic, and pathologic identification of nodes.[32]

Contrary to traditional thinking that resection of an upper pole mass necessitates resection of the adrenal gland, adrenalectomy should be reserved for patients with preoperative assessment showing direct adrenal gland involvement.[33] The incidence of adrenal gland involvement is low (1.4%) in all RCC, and routine ipsilateral adrenalectomy has not historically shown increased OS.[34,35] Although no prospective studies (to our knowledge) have explored adrenalectomy in the contemporary setting, the role of the urologist is to outweigh the survival benefits based on individual patient risk for perioperative morbidity and mortality.

Invasion of the inferior vena cava usually requires a thrombectomy in the absence of distant metastases. The surgical approach depends on thrombus characteristics of site, volume, mobility, and degree of obstruction; lower level thrombi (I and II) are feasible under simple thrombectomy, but higher level thrombi (III and IV) require a multidisciplinary team of cardiovascular and hepatobiliary experts to maneuver atrial and distal caval involvement.[36] The current evidence is based on expert consensus and retrospective case series, and the decision to resect is at the discretion of the urologist. However, stronger evidence in the form of prospective studies can reinforce guidelines in this area, especially with the advent of immunotherapy and neoadjuvant therapy.[37]

Adjuvant Therapy

Radical nephrectomy is highly effective in resecting locoregional RCC in earlier stage patients, but the 5-year risk of recurrence rate is up to 40% for stage II and III patients.[38] Postsurgical adjuvant therapy is an option to reduce disease progression, and the evidence for its use is currently controversial. The emergence of targeted therapy in metastatic RCC has paved the path for its use in adjuvant therapy, with several clinical trials exploring the efficacy and safety profiles of the same drugs. Five multicenter clinical trials have explored the use of these agents on mainly clear cell RCC subtypes, involving four TKIs (sunitinib, sorafenib, pazopanib, axitinib) and a single chimeric monoclonal antibody (girentuximab).[39–43]

- The ARISER trial (n = 864) began studying the effects of carbonic anhydrase IX chimeric monoclonal antibody, girentuximab, in an adjuvant setting.[39] This placebo-controlled phase III study yielded nonsignificant differences in disease-free survival (DFS; hazard ratio [HR], 0.97; 95% CI, 0.79–1.18) nor OS (HR, 0.99; 95% CI, 0.74–1.32). The treatment was well-tolerated by the patient population, and showed a nonsignificant DFS benefit in patients with high CAIX scores in resected tissue specimen, which prompts further investigation into adjuvant regimens guided by biomarkers from biopsy samples.

- The ASSURE trial (n = 1943) was a 3-arm trial involving both non–clear cell and clear cell subtypes, where proportionate numbers of patients were exposed to either sunitinib, sorafenib, or placebo.[40] This phase III trial showed no benefit of either sunitinib (DFS of 5.8 years; HR, 1.02; 97.5% CI, 0.85–1.23) or sorafenib (DFS of 6.1 years; HR, 0.97; 97.5% CI, 0.80–1.17) compared with placebo (DFS of 6.6 years) as adjuvant therapy, and demonstrated detrimental toxicities (eg, hypertension, fatigue, hand–foot syndrome) despite dose reduction. The results prompted a recommendation against antiangiogenic agents for adjuvant therapy. It is important to note that this trial was only 1 of the 5 discussed that includes the non–clear cell subtype (~20% of the sample size), alluding to heterogeneity of the patient groups studied.

- The recent S-TRAC trial (n = 720) explored sunitinib as an adjuvant agent for patients with high-risk clear cell subtype disease according to the UCLA Integrated Staging System criteria.[41] This trial demonstrated significant DFS improvement in the sunitinib arm (HR, 0.76; 95% CI, 0.59–0.98; P = .03), in exchange for worse adverse events compared with placebo, and the OS has yet to be reported.[44] Further S-TRAC investigations have demonstrated the predictability of the safety profile and importance of stratifying disease recurrence risk via biomarkers in sunitinib adjuvant therapy.[45,46]

- The PROTECT trial (n = 1538) investigated pazopanib compared with placebo with a starting dose of 800 mg.[42] Owing to severe adverse events, the dose reduction to 600 mg was warranted, and showed nonsignificant differences in DFS (HR, 0.86; 95% CI, 0.70–1.06) compared with placebo. Interestingly, a nondefinitive subgroup analysis of patients receiving 800 mg pazopanib showed significant DFS improvement (HR, 0.69; 95% CI, 0.51–0.94) with similar adverse event profile as a 600 mg dose.

- The most recent ATLAS trial (n = 724) showed nonsignificant differences in DFS per investigator for axitinib (TKI) intervention compared with placebo (HR, 0.870; 95% CI, 0.66–1.15). Proper DFS analysis was not possible owing to treatment discontinuations (n = 380 in total), but a subsequent subgroup analysis suggested that the highest risk patients would benefit from adjuvant therapy. Furthermore, there were more treatment-related grade 3 or 4 adverse events in the axitinib arm.

These 5 trials have failed to conclusively demonstrate the benefits of adjuvant therapy, with only the S-TRAC trial showing positive results. The variability among the results could be attributed to inherent differences in trial design, including inclusion criteria (eg, non–clear cell subtype, earlier tumor stages), risk stratification (scoring systems), and dosage manipulations. Additionally, the trials were often plagued by slow accrual and retention. Aside from these limitations, the subsequent analysis from these trials confidently suggests that proper patient selection is important for adjuvant therapy. Both S-TRAC and ATLAS trials demonstrated that higher risk patients benefit most from adjuvant therapy, and S-TRAC showed the importance of individualized tissue evaluation for targeted therapy.[41,43,46] The landscape of adjuvant therapy could shift the focus on investigating certain subgroups The ongoing clinical trials in TKIs (eg, SORCE, EVEREST) and combined-neoadjuvant therapies (eg, PROSPER, KEYNOTE-564, CheckMate 914, Immotion010) will be beneficial in confirming the optimal management in advanced locoregional RCC.

MANAGEMENT OF METASTATIC DISEASE
Cytoreductive Nephrectomies

Cytoreductive nephrectomy (CN) is radical nephrectomy performed in the presence of known metastatic disease. Optimal patient selection for CN is an area of debate among clinicians after the introduction of TKI and ICI management, because the benefits of CN must outweigh the costs of perioperative and postoperative mortality.

Perioperative morbidity may delay or preclude a patient from receiving important systemic therapy. Prospective trials before TKIs have concluded that CN is valuable for favorable-risk metastatic RCC patients before cytokine therapy, especially after careful selection for favorable prognostic factors.[47]

The emergence of TKIs triggered interest in its role in CN, with early retrospective trials showing support for CN after TKIs.[48,49] Choueiri and colleagues[48] (n = 314) explored the role of sunitinib, orafenib, and bevacizumab in CN to demonstrate significantly higher OS (19.8 months vs 9.4 months; P<.01) and independent OS benefit after adjusting for prognostic factors (HR, 0.68; 95% CI, 0.46–0.99; P<.05). A large retrospective study (n = 1658) using the International Metastatic RCC Database Consortium criteria reported higher median OS with CN (20.6 months vs 9.5 months; P<.01) and a 40% decreased risk of death after adjusting for prognostic factors (HR, 0.60; 95% CI, 0.52–0.69; P<.0001).[49] The results from retrospective trials have triggered initiation of prospective trials to solidify the role of CN in metastatic RCC management.

Recently, 2 pivotal prospective trials have challenged CN's role for metastatic RCC patients. First, the CARMENA trial (n = 450) showed sunitinib alone is noninferior to combination of sunitinib and CN based on OS (HR for death, 0.89; 95% CI, 0.71–1.10, upper boundary to noninferiority of 1.20) in intermediate- or poor-risk patients according to the Memorial Sloan Kettering Cancer Center risk score.[50] Evidence of selection bias is possible owing to the trial's slow accrual of patients from high-volume centers. Next, the SURTIME trial (n = 99) demonstrated that the timing of CN, either immediately after diagnosis or deferred after 3 cycles of sunitinib therapy, did not play a role in progression-free rate at 28 weeks (P = .61) and the median OS was not significantly higher in the deferred CN group for the per-protocol population (P = .23).[51] This outcome is interpreted as to use upfront systemic therapy to identify good responders who may benefit most from CN.

Although the current status of the use of CN remains disputed, both perspectives agree on the importance of patient selection in the decision-making progress. Current guidelines state that patients with more favorable risk should undergo CN, whereas intermediate- to poor-risk patients should undergo careful assessment to outweigh the operative consequences.[52] Some controversy remains over inclusion of time from diagnosis to treatment with systemic therapy as a prognostic risk factor that may preclude patients from receiving CN, and whether intermediate-risk candidates should be broken down into those with one prognostic factor or two. The role of CN will continue to evolve for metastatic RCC, and the use of immunomodulatory agents will be valuable in its future utilization.

Systemic Therapies

The nonsurgical nature of metastatic RCC predisposes urologists to incorporate a systemic approach in controlling the disease. Although traditionally within the field of medical oncology, urologists are increasingly participating in the prescribing and monitoring of patients on systemic therapies. A pivotal moment occurred with the newly discovered role of targeted therapies in metastatic RCC. Targeted therapy is designed to target the molecular pathways related to hallmarks of cancer growth, and can relatively isolate the therapeutic effects to the tumor itself. Two main categories of therapies are used: (1) Vascular endothelial growth factor (VEGF) inhibitors and (2) mammalian target of rapamycin (mTOR) inhibitors, which both tackle a key molecule in the hypoxia-inducing factor pathway that drive cancer progression.

The first landmark trial in 2007 (n = 750) demonstrated superior progression-free survival (PFS), ORR, and safety profile of sunitinib (VEGFR inhibitor) over the conventional interferon alpha, shifting the landscape of RCC management to consider sunitinib as a first-line treatment option.[53] Other VEGF-modulating agents, including pazopanib, cabozantinib, axitinib, sorafenib, and bevacizumab, emerged in response to failure of first-line therapy, and are considered alternative options if sunitinib is not tolerated.[54–58] The ARCC-3 trial showed clinical efficacy of mTOR inhibition, because temsirolimus showed significant improvement in OS and PFS compared with the standard interferon-alpha group, and was considered as a first-line option for poor-risk patients in a subsequent subgroup analysis.[59] Everolimus (an mTOR inhibitor) demonstrates prolonged survival as a second-line treatment plan after failure of VEGF pathway therapy.[60] The emergence of targeted therapy has provided more weapons to manage metastatic RCC as a first-line therapy, and continued clinical trials have attempted to optimize treatment plans. Currently, the use of VEGF and mTOR inhibitors are limited to second-line therapy (especially cabozanitib) and as alternative options owing to the advent of ICIs.[13]

The landscape of metastatic RCC management has undergone a retrograde shift back to immunotherapy with promising development involving ICIs. Unlike cytokines, ICIs are monoclonal antibodies that target specific T-cell interactions suppressed by tumors. Combination therapy is the standard approach with the use of ICIs. ICIs include (1) PD-1 and PD-L1 inhibitors (opposite ligand arm of PD-1), and (2) cytotoxic T-lymphocyte associated protein 4 inhibitors. The emergence of ICIs began with promising results from Checkmate 025 phase III trial in 2015 (n = 821) that demonstrated improvement in OS for nivolumab (a PD-1 inhibitor) monotherapy versus everolimus.[61]

After nivolumab's success, there was a great deal of interest in tackling multiple arms of the immune response in the form of combination therapies. Ipilimumab (cytotoxic T-lymphocyte associated protein-4 inhibitor) was first used in advanced melanoma, and is now been used in the management of metastatic RCC in combination with nivolumab. The milestone Checkmate 214 trial (n = 847) demonstrated an improvement of the nivolumab-ipilimumab combination over sunitinib in OS (HR for death, 0.63; 99.8% CI, 0.44–0.89; $P<.001$), ORR (42% vs 27%; $P<.001$), and a more favorable safety profile (lower incidence of grade 3 and 4 related adverse events) in intermediate- and poor-risk patient groups.[62] This therapy is now suggested to be the new standard first-line therapy for intermediate- to poor-risk patients.

The successes of ICI dual therapy motivated clinical trials to combine ICI with other antitumor agents, including VEGF inhibitors. The focus has been on tumors with positive PD-L1 expression, which will be the main target for ICIs on the tumor surface. Atezolizumab (PD-L1 inhibitor) plus bevacizumab (VEGF inhibitor) in the pivotal Immotion 151 phase III trial (n = 915) demonstrated improvements in OS (11.2 months vs 7.7 months; HR, 0.74; 95% CI, 0.57–0.96; $P = .02$) over sunitinib in a PD-L1–positive population at interim analysis with a more favorable safety profile.[63] The atezolimumab plus bevacizumab group also demonstrated higher ORR and complete response rate compared with the sunitinib group (ORR, 37% vs 33%; complete response rate, 5% vs 3%). The PD-L1–positive group is the only group that yielded significant results from this trial, which prompts further investigation into biomarkers but is less immediately relevant in the clinical context.

The KEYNOTE-426 trial (n = 861) demonstrated that the pembrolizumab (PD-1 inhibitor) and axitinib (VEGFR inhibitor) combination was superior to sunitinib in PFS (15.1 months vs 11.1 months; HR, 0.69; 95% CI, 0.57–0.84; $P<.001$) in the intention-to-treat population.[64] The benefits to OS were demonstrated across all International Metastatic RCC Database Consortium groups and between PD-L1 expression groups. Moreover, the ORR was significantly higher in the pembrolizumab plus axitinib group (59.3% vs 35.7%; $P<.001$) with higher complete response rates (5.8% vs 1.9%). This trial demonstrated the superiority of pembrolizumab plus axitinib over sunitinib in most endpoints, with the exception of safety profile, which showed unexpected adverse events for the combination therapy group, such as elevated liver enzymes.

Finally, the avelumab (a PD-L1 inhibitor) plus axitinib (a VEGF inhibitor) combination in the JAVELIN Renal 101 trial (n = 886) resulted in significant PFS improvement in the PD-L1–positive population (13.8 months vs 7.2 months; HR, 0.61; 95% CI, 0.47–0.79; $P<.001$), as well as the overall population (13.8 months vs 8.4 months; HR, 0.69; 95% CI, 0.56–0.84; $P<.001$).[65] Although the OS data are not mature, the avelumab plus axitinib combination shows promising clinical efficacy, because the ORRs are double in comparison with sunitinib in the PD-L1–positive population (55.2% vs 25.5%) and the overall population (51.4% vs 25.7%).

Combination immunotherapies have shown promising results in most end points compared with sunitinib, and these results will be reflected in future guidelines of metastatic RCC management. A recent Canadian guideline has established these options as preferred first-line therapy for treatment-naïve patients with metastatic RCC in all risk groups.[13] Moreover, the results suggest the superiority of these therapies despite biomarker selection, because PD-L1 expression status was not necessary to benefit from these drug regimes, especially for pembrolizumb plus axitinib and avelumab plus axitinib. Currently, there are many clinical trials exploring the use of other combinations of antitumor agents.[66]

Despite promising clinical trial results, as a clinician, it is difficult to ignore the adverse events associated with these newer agents. TKIs are used frequently in managing late stage RCC, but are associated with myriad adverse events, and grade 3 and 4 toxicities are not uncommon.[67] The main clinical response would be symptomatic management through additional medications and TKI dosage reduction, but adds concern for contraindication and diminished efficacy, respectively. The more recent ICIs are associated with a unique group of toxicities called immune-related adverse events that could be stabilized using steroid therapy or treatment discontinuation.[4] Patient quality of life is an important consideration for any therapy, and future clinical trials can optimize treatment to maintain drug response and minimize adverse events. Currently, the urologist's role is to carefully assess and regularly follow-up with patients under systemic therapy to recognize secondary medical conditions and treat necessary adverse events based on clinical judgment.

Oral formulations of TKIs and mTOR inhibitors have facilitated outpatient management that can be done in the hands of an experienced urologist familiar with their indications and toxicities. Patients in our clinic are seen on a regular basis with routine bloodwork and dose adjustments overseen by urologists with intermittent reimaging every 3 to 6 months to assess for radiologic response or progression. The intravenous formulation of ICIs has necessitated that they be administered through our local cancer center in conjunction with medical oncologists who can manage the associated toxicities. As our experience with these newer agents grows, there may be an increased role for urologists in this setting.

SUMMARY

Since the advent of targeted therapies for advanced RCC, urologists have become more involved in the care of patients at all stages of disease. TKIs have demonstrated improved survival at a population level and ICIs are under investigation as the next agents of choice for advanced RCC. TKIs and ICIs are easier to administer and monitor compared with traditional chemotherapeutic agents and are largely being incorporated into urology practice. The promising results of ICIs provides impetus for more clinical trials to develop safer and more efficacious drug regimens for tackling advanced kidney cancer. Furthermore, the role of surgery in advanced RCC is shifting with increased targeted therapy with trials continuing to understand CN and other complex surgeries. The next direction for RCC research will be to individualize treatments by identifying biomarkers within tumors that can aid in prognosis and treatment recommendations to ensure optimal responses and safety profiles. The role of the urologist in treating advanced RCC has expanded beyond the surgical realm, and the recent advancements in the field will enhance the ability to treat these patients at all stages of disease.

DISCLOSURE

The authors have no conflicts of interest to declare.

REFERENCES

1. Bray F, Ferlay J, Soerjomataram I, et al. Global cancer statistics 2018: GLOBOCAN estimates of incidence and mortality worldwide for 36 cancers in 185 countries. CA Cancer J Clin 2018;68(6): 394–424.

2. Capitanio U, Bensalah K, Bex A, et al. Epidemiology of renal cell carcinoma. Eur Urol 2019;75(1):74–84.

3. Capitanio U, Montorsi F. Renal cancer. Lancet 2016; 387(10021):894–906.

4. Grimm M-O, Bex A, De Santis M, et al. Safe Use of Immune Checkpoint Inhibitors in the Multidisciplinary Management of Urological Cancer: the European Association of Urology Position in 2019. Eur Urol 2019;76(3):368–80.

5. Siddiqui SA, Frank I, Leibovich BC, et al. Impact of tumor size on the predictive ability of the pT3a primary tumor classification for renal cell carcinoma. J Urol 2007;177(1):59–62.

6. Keegan KA, Schupp CW, Chamie K, et al. Histopathology of surgically treated renal cell carcinoma: survival differences by subtype and stage. J Urol 2012;188(2):391–7.

7. Klatte T, Rossi SH, Stewart GD. Prognostic factors and prognostic models for renal cell carcinoma: a literature review. World J Urol 2018;36(12):1943–52.

8. Heng DYC, Xie W, Regan MM, et al. External validation and comparison with other models of the International Metastatic Renal-Cell Carcinoma Database Consortium prognostic model: a population-based study. Lancet Oncol 2013;14(2):141–8.

9. Maloni R, Lavallée LT, McAlpine K, et al. Kidney Cancer Research Network of Canada (KCRNC) consensus statement on the role of renal mass biopsy in the management of kidney cancer. Can Urol Assoc J 2019;13(12):377–83.

10. Volpe A, Finelli A, Gill IS, et al. Rationale for percutaneous biopsy and histologic characterisation of renal tumours. Eur Urol 2012;62(3):491–504.

11. Tannir NM, Jonasch E, Albiges L, et al. Everolimus Versus Sunitinib Prospective Evaluation in Metastatic Non–Clear Cell Renal Cell Carcinoma (ESPN): a randomized multicenter phase 2 trial. Eur Urol 2016;69(5):866–74.

12. Armstrong AJ, Halabi S, Eisen T, et al. Everolimus versus sunitinib for patients with metastatic non-clear cell renal cell carcinoma (ASPEN): a multicentre, open-label, randomised phase 2 trial. Lancet Oncol 2016;17(3):378–88.

13. Hotte SJ, Kapoor A, Basappa NS, et al. Management of advanced kidney cancer: Kidney Cancer Research Network of Canada (KCRNC) consensus update 2019. Can Urol Assoc J 2019;13(10):343–54.

14. Manley BJ, Hakimi AA. Molecular profiling of renal cell carcinoma: building a bridge toward clinical impact. Curr Opin Urol 2016;26(5):383–7.

15. Rhoades Smith KE, Bilen MA. A review of papillary renal cell carcinoma and MET inhibitors. Kidney cancer 2019;3(3):151–61.

16. Marconi L, Dabestani S, Lam TB, et al. Systematic review and meta-analysis of diagnostic accuracy of percutaneous renal tumour biopsy. Eur Urol 2016;69(4):660–73.

17. Bindayi A, Hamilton ZA, McDonald ML, et al. Neoadjuvant therapy for localized and locally advanced renal cell carcinoma. Urol Oncol Semin Orig Investig 2018;36(1):31–7.

18. Silberstein JL, Millard F, Mehrazin R, et al. Feasibility and efficacy of neoadjuvant sunitinib before nephron-sparing surgery. BJU Int 2010;106(9): 1270–6.

19. Hellenthal NJ, Underwood W, Penetrante R, et al. Prospective clinical trial of preoperative sunitinib in patients with renal cell carcinoma. J Urol 2010; 184(3):859–64.

20. Rini BI, Plimack ER, Takagi T, et al. A Phase II Study of Pazopanib in Patients with Localized Renal Cell Carcinoma to Optimize Preservation of Renal Parenchyma. J Urol 2015;194(2):297–303.

21. Lane BR, Derweesh IH, Kim HL, et al. Presurgical sunitinib reduces tumor size and may facilitate partial nephrectomy in patients with renal cell carcinoma. Urol Oncol Semin Orig Investig 2015;33(3): 112.e15–21.

22. Zhang Y, Li Y, Deng J, et al. Sorafenib neoadjuvant therapy in the treatment of high risk renal cell carcinoma. Dahiya R, editor. PLoS One 2015;10(2): e0115896.

23. Karam JA, Devine CE, Urbauer DL, et al. Phase 2 trial of neoadjuvant axitinib in patients with locally advanced nonmetastatic clear cell renal cell carcinoma. Eur Urol 2014;66(5):874–80.

24. McCormick B, Meissner MA, Karam JA, et al. Surgical complications of presurgical systemic therapy for renal cell carcinoma: a systematic review. Kidney cancer 2017;1(2):115–21.

25. Cost NG, Delacroix SE, Sleeper JP, et al. The impact of targeted molecular therapies on the level of renal cell carcinoma vena caval tumor thrombus. Eur Urol 2011;59(6):912–8.

26. Gill IS, Kavoussi LR, Lane BR, et al. Comparison of 1,800 laparoscopic and open partial nephrectomies for single renal tumors. J Urol 2007;178(1):41–6.

27. Shapiro E, Benway BM, Wang AJ, et al. The role of nephron-sparing robotic surgery in the management of renal malignancy. Curr Opin Urol 2009;19(1): 76–80.

28. Burgess NA, Koo BC, Calvert RC, et al. Randomized trial of laparoscopic v open nephrectomy. J Endourol 2007;21(6):610–3.

29. Bekema HJ, MacLennan S, Imamura M, et al. Systematic review of adrenalectomy and lymph node dissection in locally advanced renal cell carcinoma. Eur Urol 2013;64(5):799–810.

30. Blom JHM, van Poppel H, Maréchal JM, et al. Radical nephrectomy with and without lymph-node dissection: final results of European Organization for Research and Treatment of Cancer (EORTC) randomized phase 3 trial 30881. Eur Urol 2009;55(1): 28–34.

31. Gershman B, Thompson RH, Boorjian SA, et al. Radical nephrectomy with or without lymph node dissection for high risk nonmetastatic renal cell carcinoma: a multi-institutional analysis. J Urol 2018; 199(5):1143–8.

32. Zareba P, Pinthus JH, Russo P. The contemporary role of lymph node dissection in the management of renal cell carcinoma. Ther Adv Urol 2018;10(11): 335–42.

33. Rendon RA, Kapoor A, Breau R, et al. Surgical management of renal cell carcinoma: Canadian Kidney Cancer Forum Consensus. Can Urol Assoc J 2014; 8(5–6):E398–412.

34. Weight CJ, Kim SP, Lohse CM, et al. Routine adrenalectomy in patients with locally advanced renal cell cancer does not offer oncologic benefit and places a significant portion of patients at risk for an asynchronous metastasis in a solitary adrenal gland. Eur Urol 2011;60(3):458–64.

35. Yap SA, Alibhai SM, Abouassally R, et al. Do we continue to unnecessarily perform ipsilateral adrenalectomy at the time of radical nephrectomy? A population based study. J Urol 2012;187(2): 398–404.

36. Manassero F, Mogorovich A, Di Paola G, et al. Renal cell carcinoma with caval involvement: contemporary strategies of surgical treatment. Urol Oncol 2011;29(6):745–50.

37. Lardas M, Stewart F, Scrimgeour D, et al. Systematic review of surgical management of nonmetastatic renal cell carcinoma with vena caval thrombus. Eur Urol 2016;70(2):265–80.

38. Janowitz T, Welsh SJ, Zaki K, et al. Adjuvant therapy in renal cell carcinoma—past, present, and future. Semin Oncol 2013;40(4):482–91.

39. Chamie K, Donin NM, Klöpfer P, et al. Adjuvant weekly girentuximab following nephrectomy for high-risk renal cell carcinoma. JAMA Oncol 2017; 3(7):913.

40. Haas NB, Manola J, Uzzo RG, et al. Adjuvant sunitinib or sorafenib for high-risk, non-metastatic renal-cell carcinoma (ECOG-ACRIN E2805): a double-blind, placebo-controlled, randomised, phase 3 trial. Lancet 2016;387(10032):2008–16.

41. Ravaud A, Motzer RJ, Pandha HS, et al. Adjuvant sunitinib in high-risk renal-cell carcinoma after nephrectomy. N Engl J Med 2016;375(23):2246–54.

42. Motzer RJ, Haas NB, Donskov F, et al. Randomized phase III trial of adjuvant pazopanib versus placebo after nephrectomy in patients with localized or locally advanced renal cell carcinoma. J Clin Oncol 2017;35(35):3916–23.

43. Gross-Goupil M, Kwon TG, Eto M, et al. Axitinib versus placebo as an adjuvant treatment of renal cell carcinoma: results from the phase III, randomized ATLAS trial. Ann Oncol 2018;29(12):2371–8.

44. Motzer RJ, Ravaud A, Patard J-J, et al. Adjuvant sunitinib for high-risk renal cell carcinoma after nephrectomy: subgroup analyses and updated overall survival results. Eur Urol 2018;73(1):62–8.

45. Staehler M, Motzer RJ, George DJ, et al. Adjuvant sunitinib in patients with high-risk renal cell carcinoma: safety, therapy management, and patient-reported outcomes in the S-TRAC trial. Ann Oncol 2018;29(10):2098–104.

46. Rini BI, Escudier B, Martini J-F, et al. Validation of the 16-gene recurrence score in patients with locoregional, high-risk renal cell carcinoma from a phase III trial of adjuvant sunitinib. Clin Cancer Res 2018; 24(18):4407–15.

47. Flanigan RC, Mickisch G, Sylvester R, et al. Cytoreductive nephrectomy in patients with metastatic renal cancer: a combined analysis. J Urol 2004; 171(3):1071–6.

48. Choueiri TK, Xie W, Kollmannsberger C, et al. The impact of cytoreductive nephrectomy on survival of patients with metastatic renal cell carcinoma receiving vascular endothelial growth factor targeted therapy. J Urol 2011;185(1):60–6.

49. Heng DYC, Wells JC, Rini BI, et al. Cytoreductive nephrectomy in patients with synchronous metastases from renal cell carcinoma: results from the international metastatic renal cell carcinoma database consortium. Eur Urol 2014;66(4):704–10.

50. Méjean A, Ravaud A, Thezenas S, et al. Sunitinib alone or after nephrectomy in metastatic renal-cell carcinoma. N Engl J Med 2018;379(5):417–27.

51. Bex A, Mulders P, Jewett M, et al. Comparison of immediate vs deferred cytoreductive nephrectomy in patients with synchronous metastatic renal cell carcinoma receiving sunitinib. JAMA Oncol 2019;5(2): 164.

52. Mason RJ, Wood L, Kapoor A, et al. Kidney Cancer Research Network of Canada (KCRNC) consensus statement on the role of cytoreductive nephrectomy for patients with metastatic renal cell carcinoma. Can Urol Assoc J 2019;13(6):166–74.

53. Motzer RJ, Hutson TE, Tomczak P, et al. Sunitinib versus interferon alfa in metastatic renal-cell carcinoma. N Engl J Med 2007;356(2):115–24.

54. Motzer RJ, Hutson TE, Cella D, et al. Pazopanib versus sunitinib in metastatic renal-cell carcinoma. N Engl J Med 2013;369(8):722–31.

55. Choueiri TK, Halabi S, Sanford BL, et al. Cabozantinib versus sunitinib as initial targeted therapy for patients with metastatic renal cell carcinoma of poor or intermediate risk: the alliance A031203 CABOSUN trial. J Clin Oncol 2017;35(6):591–7.

56. Rini BI, Escudier B, Tomczak P, et al. Comparative effectiveness of axitinib versus sorafenib in advanced renal cell carcinoma (AXIS): a randomised phase 3 trial. Lancet 2011;378(9807):1931–9.

57. Escudier B, Eisen T, Stadler WM, et al. Sorafenib in advanced clear-cell renal-cell carcinoma. N Engl J Med 2007;356(2):125–34.

58. Escudier B, Pluzanska A, Koralewski P, et al. Bevacizumab plus interferon alfa-2a for treatment of metastatic renal cell carcinoma: a randomised, double-blind phase III trial. Lancet 2007;370(9605): 2103–11.

59. Hudes G, Carducci M, Tomczak P, et al. Temsirolimus, interferon alfa, or both for advanced renal-cell carcinoma. N Engl J Med 2007;356(22): 2271–81.

60. Motzer RJ, Escudier B, Oudard S, et al. Efficacy of everolimus in advanced renal cell carcinoma: a double-blind, randomised, placebo-controlled phase III trial. Lancet 2008;372(9637):449–56.

61. Motzer RJ, Escudier B, McDermott DF, et al. Nivolumab versus Everolimus in advanced renal-cell carcinoma. N Engl J Med 2015;373(19):1803–13.

62. Motzer RJ, Tannir NM, McDermott DF, et al. Nivolumab plus Ipilimumab versus Sunitinib in advanced renal-cell carcinoma. N Engl J Med 2018;378(14): 1277–90.

63. Rini BI, Powles T, Atkins MB, et al. Atezolizumab plus bevacizumab versus sunitinib in patients with previously untreated metastatic renal cell carcinoma (IMmotion151): a multicentre, open-label, phase 3, randomised controlled trial. Lancet 2019; 393(10189):2404–15.

64. Rini BI, Plimack ER, Stus V, et al. Pembrolizumab plus Axitinib versus Sunitinib for advanced renal-cell carcinoma. N Engl J Med 2019;380(12): 1116–27.

65. Motzer RJ, Penkov K, Haanen J, et al. Avelumab plus Axitinib versus Sunitinib for advanced renal-cell carcinoma. N Engl J Med 2019;380(12): 1103–15.

66. Flippot R, Escudier B, Albiges L. Immune checkpoint inhibitors: toward new paradigms in renal cell carcinoma. Drugs 2018;78(14):1443–57.

67. Di Lorenzo G, Porta C, Bellmunt J, et al. Toxicities of targeted therapy and their management in kidney cancer. Eur Urol 2011;59(4):526–40.

Imaging for Metastatic Renal Cell Carcinoma

Soumya V.L. Vig, MD[a], Elcin Zan, MD[a], Stella K. Kang, MD, MSc[a,b,*]

KEYWORDS

- Metastatic disease • Renal cell carcinoma • MRI • CT • PET

KEY POINTS

- Imaging modalities for metastatic renal cell carcinoma offer synergistic soft tissue characterization for staging evaluation.
- Clinical suspicion for osseous or central nervous system metastasis remains the recommended driver for imaging specific to these organ systems.
- Imaging criteria for tumor assessment during systemic therapy and for likelihood of response to first-line antiangiogenic agents may need to account for markers of vascularity rather than size alone for prognostication.

INTRODUCTION

Renal cell carcinoma (RCC) accounts for approximately 5% of adult cases of cancer in men and 3% in women and is the second most common urologic neoplasm found in both sexes.[1] Approximately 33% to 50% of patients have metastatic disease at the time of detection.[2] In addition, 20% to 40% of patients with RCC develop metastatic disease after radical nephrectomy.[3,4] Approximately 25% to 50% of those treated for localized disease develop metastatic disease.[2] Monitoring for metastatic disease development and progression relies mostly on imaging. The increasing use of diagnostic imaging has resulted in tumors being diagnosed incidentally at an earlier stage and smaller size, but dedicated staging protocols may still be needed to provide accurate staging evaluation once RCC is suspected.[5] The stage of disease is the most important factor in determining prognosis and determining the risk of relapse.

Imaging plays a key role in surveillance and assessment of treatment response after the diagnosis of metastatic disease by aiding clinicians in tailoring treatments.[3] Systemic therapies for metastatic RCC have evolved from the earliest forms in the 1980s based on adoptive immunotherapy. By the early 1990s, interleukin-2, interferon, or a combination of the two were widely adopted.[6] Immunotherapy with interferon or interleukin-2 was the standard of care, but with response rates of only 10% to 20%.[3,7] However, with newer agents, such as tyrosine kinase inhibitors, patients have partial response rates of 4% to 40% and more than 75% demonstrate minor response or stabilization of disease.[8] Randomized trials have also shown promising results with vascular endothelial growth factor inhibitors and anti–programmed death ligand in molecular targeted therapies.[9,10] With such treatment advances, imaging evaluation of response may play an increasingly crucial role in decision-making about available systemic therapies. This review article provides updates on the role of imaging in metastatic RCC and describes newer techniques under investigation for staging and treatment response.

[a] Department of Radiology, NYU Langone Medical Center, New York, NY 10016, USA; [b] Department of Population Health NYU Langone Medical Center, New York, NY 10016, USA
* Corresponding author. Department of Radiology, NYU Langone Medical Center, 660 First Avenue, Room 333, New York, NY 10016.
E-mail address: stella.kang@nyulangone.org

Urol Clin N Am 47 (2020) 281–291
https://doi.org/10.1016/j.ucl.2020.04.005

ROLE OF DIAGNOSTIC RADIOLOGY IN EVALUATION FOR METASTATIC DISEASE: COMPUTED TOMOGRAPHY AND MRI

Abdominal computed tomography (CT) and MRI are the mainstay of staging the primary tumor at initial diagnosis, including evaluation for locoregional nodal or abdominal visceral metastases.[11] Protocols are designed to fully evaluate the extent of the primary tumor and for metastatic RCC. The recommended CT technique for the initial staging evaluation includes arterial and nephrographic/portal venous phases to identify hypervascular tumors and also delineate arterial and venous structures.[11] Imaging is acquired at 15 to 30 and 80 to 90, seconds, respectively, to capture these phases.

Clear cell carcinoma is the most common subtype of RCC and demonstrates avid arterial enhancement as opposed to papillary or chromophobe subtypes (**Fig. 1**). These differences are related to intratumoral vascularity. Therefore, clear cell metastases generally also demonstrate avid arterial enhancement and can be undetectable in nephrographic phases.[1] However, non–clear cell subtypes may enhance to a lesser degree and are better detected on nephrographic phases.[1] The nephrographic/portal venous phase is used to evaluate the venous system to evaluate for invasion and/or surgical planning. Additional delayed

excretory phase images, captured at 180 seconds, can also be obtained if there is concern for extension into the collecting system.[11] Excretory images are helpful in detecting identifying filling defects in the ureters and can supplement routine surveillance when there is a clinical concern. Other helpful study components include multiplanar reformatted images and three-dimensional volume-rendered images, with the latter helpful in visualization of the relationships of structures for preoperative planning. In addition, these images can help assess tumor stage, delineating the tumor with particular attention to the relationship of the tumor to adjacent structures, including vascular relationships.[11] Such reformations are best obtained with the thinnest possible images (typically <1.5-mm interval and 10%–50% overlap).[11]

MRI is generally used when iodinated contrast is contraindicated or when further characterization of soft tissue is needed to determine disease extent. For MRI, protocols should include gadolinium-enhanced and noncontrast T1 sequences.[12] Just as in CT, arterial phase imaging is useful in detection of clear cell type metastases. For example, one can see an avidly arterially enhancing focus in the left adrenal gland, which was biopsy proven as metastatic clear cell RCC. Arterial phase imaging can be used in initial staging and recurrence as commonly done with CT; tumor proximity

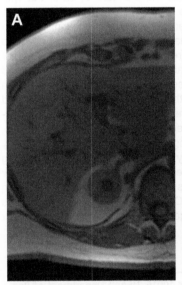 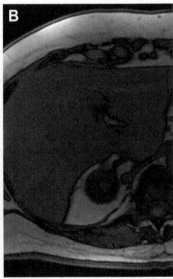 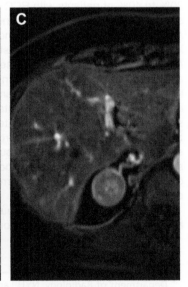

Fig. 1. Adrenal collision tumor with clear cell RCC. A 69-year-old man with history of left clear cell RCC status postnephrectomy in 1987. He was found to have a right adrenal adenoma. T1-weighted in-phase (*A*) and out-of-phase (*B*) sequences demonstrate loss of signal on out-of-phase images, suggestive of microscopic fat as seen in adrenal adenomas. However, a central portion demonstrates India ink artifact, suggesting an interface of fat with nonfatty soft tissue. The center also avidly enhances on postcontrast imaging (*C*), suggesting metastasis. Pathology confirmed adrenal adenoma containing metastatic RCC.

vasculature is important in surgical planning. Other useful sequences in MRI can also help identify RCC metastases. For example, diffusion weighting is used to more easily identify lymph nodes in the retroperitoneum, which may be less conspicuous on other sequences; use of diffusion-weighted imaging can increase sensitivity to detect smaller lymph nodes and those that may have less contrast to abutting structures.[13] RCC are cellular tumors that demonstrate diffusion restriction.[13] In addition, they contain intravoxel fat, which occasionally is seen in metastasis. Papillary subtype to be specific may not demonstrate avid arterial enhancement but demonstrates diffusion restriction.[13] Therefore, diffusion imaging aids in the detection of metastatic non–clear cell subtype RCC.

RCC typically metastasizes to the lung, bone, lymph nodes, liver, adrenal glands, and brain.[1] More rare sites include skeletal muscle, bowel, gallbladder, pancreas, and orbits (**Fig. 2**). Depending on the organ system in which the metastasis may be suspected clinically, various imaging modalities are superior to others in detecting metastasis. CT and MRI play critical but distinctive roles in detection and surveillance of metastatic RCC. Guidelines slightly vary among the American Urologic Association (AUA), European Association

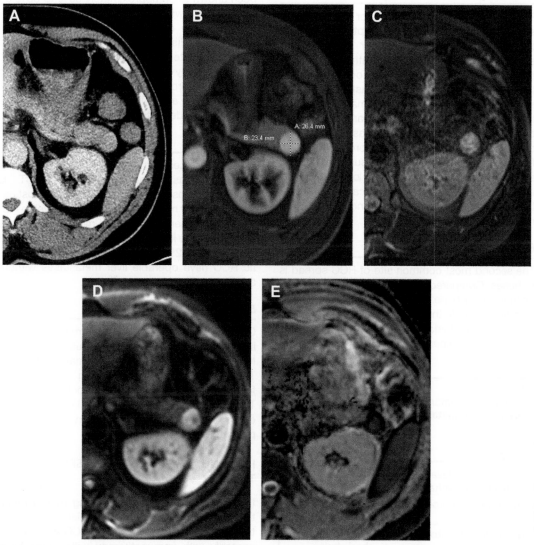

Fig. 2. Pancreatic metastasis. Patient with history of RCC was found to have a growing pancreatic tail mass on routine CT of the abdomen and pelvis. The mass enhances avidly on arterial phase images on CT (*A*) and arterial phase on MRI (*B*). On MRI, the lesion is T2 hyperintense to surrounding tissue on T2-weighted fat-saturated images (*C*). Diffusion restriction entails high signal on high b value images (*D*) and low signal on the ADC map (*E*).

of Urology, and National Comprehensive Cancer Network. AUA defines certain symptoms that should be followed by specific imaging.[8] However, the European Association of Urology and National Comprehensive Cancer Network make general recommendations, stating that bone scan, brain CT, or MRI may be used in the presence of specific clinical or laboratory signs and symptoms (Table 1).[14,15] The AUA also recommends specific time intervals for surveillance for metastatic disease based on the TNM stage of disease at presentation (Table 2).[15]

ORGAN-SPECIFIC EVALUATION FOR METASTASIS
Pulmonary

Pulmonary metastases account for 45% of metastatic RCC and are usually asymptomatic.[1] Controversies exist as to whether and how to evaluate for the possibility of intrathoracic metastases based on stage of tumors. For small primary tumors (T1), where the risk of metastatic disease is small, simple chest radiography may be satisfactory. For stage T2 or higher primary tumors, and because small pulmonary metastases are missed on radiographs, chest CT should probably be performed.[11,16] Lesions on CT are usually small, well circumscribed, and in subpleural locations. However, in RCC, patients can have "cannonball" metastases that are large (>5 cm) rounded pulmonary metastases.[1]

Bone

The second most common site of RCC spread is to bones. Compared with other malignancies, the distribution of bone metastases varies and common sites include the pelvis, spine, and ribs. Solitary bone metastases are rare.[1] For bone metastases, compared with CT, MRI is useful in

Table 1
Imaging recommendations based on clinical suspicion for metastatic RCC

Symptom	Imaging Modality Recommended
Bone pain or elevated alkaline phosphatase	Bone scan
Pulmonary symptoms	Chest radiograph or CT chest
Neurologic symptoms	CT or MRI of the brain/spine

Data from Campbell S., Uzzo R G., Allaf M E., et al., Renal Mass and Localized Renal Cancer: AUA Guideline. J Urol., 2017. 198(3); p. 520-529.

detecting smaller lesions and lesions adjacent to the bones.[16] Bone scan is recommended for patients with bone pain or elevated increased alkaline phosphatase (Fig. 3).[17]

Lymph Nodes

Lymph node metastases are the third most common site of metastasis in RCC, accounting for 22% of cases. Diagnosis of lymph node involvement is based on morphologic criteria, especially size increase seen at CT (discussed later). Both CT and MRI are equally adequate in identifying metastatic lymph nodes; however, CT is generally the mainstay in assessing lymph node sizes and locations. Staging accuracy of lymph nodes has been shown to be approximately 83% to 88% on CT and MRI, without difference between modalities, although a head-to-head comparison has not been published.[3] PET has shown moderate ability to detect lymph node metastases in RCC[18]; a study by Kang and colleagues[19] found that 18F-fluorodeoxyglucose (FDG)-PET was 75% sensitive and 100% specific for retroperitoneal lymph node metastases.

Liver

Liver metastases carry poor prognosis and multiphase contrast-enhanced abdominal CT is preferred in most surveillance regimens.[2] Most patients with liver metastases from RCC develop metastases in other locations; the metastatic disease is limited to the liver in only a small portion of these patients. Only 2% to 4% of patients with metastatic RCC have operable liver metastases without additional sites of disease.[20]

Brain

Given the low incidence of brain metastases, the literature does not support the routine use of CT/MRI or bone scans for asymptomatic patients.[16] The AUA recommends reserving brain imaging for only those who have neurologic symptoms. To date, there are no standardized imaging protocols for screening the central nervous system in patients with metastatic RCC.[17]

IMAGING ASSESSMENT TO RESPONSE TO THERAPY

Imaging has played an increasing role in monitoring response to treatment in patients on chemotherapy. Previously, metastatic RCC was treated primarily with immunotherapy with interleukin-β and interferon-α; however, the mainstay has now become antiangiogenic agents and combination with immune check point inhibitors.[21] On CT,

Table 2
The American Urologic Association categorizes follow-up imaging recommendations based on risk criteria

Low Risk (pT1N0Nx)	Moderate/High Risk (pT2-pT4 N0, Nx, or Any Stage N+)
Baseline abdominal scan (CT or MRI) for nephron-sparing surgery and abdominal imaging (US, CT, or MRI) for radical nephrectomy within 3–12 mo after surgery	Moderate- to high-risk patients are recommended to have a baseline chest and abdominal scan (CT or MRI) within 3–6 mo following surgery with continued imaging (US, CXR, CT, or MRI) every 6 mo for at least 3 y and yearly thereafter to year 5
Additional abdominal imaging (US, CT, or MRI) may be performed in patients with low-risk disease following a radical nephrectomy if the initial postoperative baseline image is negative	Site-specific imaging may be performed if clinical symptoms are suggestive of recurrence or metastatic spread
Abdominal imaging (US, CT, or MRI) may be performed annually for 3 y in patients with low-risk disease following a partial nephrectomy based on individual risk factors if the initial postoperative scan is negative	In moderate- to high-risk patients, imaging (US, CXR, CT, or MRI) beyond 5 y may be performed at the discretion of the clinician
Those with history of low-risk RCC are recommended to have annual CXR to assess for pulmonary metastases for 3 y and only as clinically indicated beyond that time period	Routine FDG-PET scan is not indicated in the follow-up for RCC

Abbreviations: CXR, chest radiograph; US, ultrasound.
Data from Campbell S., Uzzo R G., Allaf M E., et al., Renal Mass and Localized Renal Cancer: AUA Guideline. J Urol., 2017. 198(3); p. 520-529.

successful treatment is seen as diminished vascularity, attenuation and enhancement, and size; therefore, attenuation and size should be used as criteria for assessment of response to treatment.[12] Frequency and duration of follow-up imaging is not yet standardized, although a schedule of contrast-enhanced CT scans every 3 months has been reported.[12] Because of the increasing use of imaging in monitoring treatment response, various criteria have been developed over the years to help clinicians in treatment plans (**Table 3**).

Since the initial introduction of Response Evaluation Criteria in Solid Tumors (RECIST) in 2000, RECIST has been widely adopted and applied by the oncology and radiology communities to define response to treatment in clinical trials. It was created to assess objective changes in tumor size as affected by therapy and to compare the changes to tumor from future therapies with current standards of care. In 2009, the revised RECIST 1.1 guidelines were formed to simplify, optimize, and further standardize assessments of tumor burden and became the most widely used method for assessing treatment response.[22] In particular, these guidelines were more applicable to antiangiogenic agents, because the RECIST 1.0 system was originally created to assess response to cytotoxic agents.[23,24] The RECIST 1.1 criteria were based on one-dimension measurements to quantify changes in tumor size, obtained by summing the longest diameters of the target lesions in the axial plane.[1] Lesion response is classified using four categories: (1) partial, (2) progressive, (3) stable, and (4) complete response. Partial response is defined as 30% decrease in sum of the longest diameters of the target lesions. Progressive disease is defined as at least 20% increase in the sum of the longest diameters of the target lesions. Complete response is defined as disappearance of all target lesions and any pathologic lymph nodes must have reduction in short axis of less than 10 mm. Stable disease is considered when there is neither sufficient decrease to qualify for partial response nor sufficient increase to qualify for progressive disease. Thus, limitations of RECIST 1.1 stem from changes in size being better attuned to assess tumor response to cytotoxic agents. RECIST does not consider other features, such as tumor attenuation, and underestimates the response of malignancies to cytostatic therapies, such as antiangiogenic agents.[23]

Choi proposed updated criteria that incorporated some of the limitations of RECIST. Choi

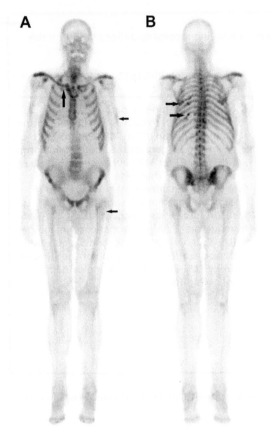

Fig. 3. Bone scan of diffuse metastatic RCC. A 68-year-old man with history of metastatic RCC, clear cell type, had a right nephrectomy in 1986. A subsequent cancer was discovered in the contralateral kidney and treated with partial nephrectomy in 2012, later requiring a complete nephrectomy because of recurrence. The patient later developed metastasis to lymph nodes, liver, and bone. A bone scan was performed to assess the metastatic disease. (A) Focal uptake represents metastases of the axial skeleton, upper and lower extremities (arrows), and (B) metastatic lesions in the ribs (arrows). The patient is status post bilateral nephrectomy with no visualization of kidneys or bladder uptake.

criteria were initially developed to assess the efficacy of using imatinib to treat gastrointestinal stromal tumors.[25,26] It was the first classification to use tumor attenuation measurements (in Hounsfield Units). Partial response was defined as greater than or equal to 10% decrease in tumor size or greater than or equal to 15% decrease in tumor attenuation in the portal phase with the region of interest placed surrounding the entire lesion. Progression was defined as greater than or equal to 10% increase in tumor size without taking tumor attenuation into account. A study done with sunitinib validated the Choi criteria, having a

significantly better predictive value for overall survival over RECIST 1.1.[23]

In 2010, Nathan and colleagues[1] proposed a combined assessment of size and arterial phase attenuation of target lesions in patients with metastatic RCC and developed the modified Choi criteria. It compared data with Choi and RECIST 1.1 and found the modified Choi to be a better predictor of clinical response, as defined by time to progression and survival in patients with metastatic RCC.

Smith and colleagues[27] proposed the Size and Attenuation CT (SACT) criteria, which like the modified Choi criteria evaluated changes in tumor size and attenuation, and also defined specific patterns of contrast enhancement in target lesions that were indicative of disease progression. Changes from central necrosis to nearly complete central enhancement were described. The proposed SACT criteria were able to stratify patients with progression-free survival greater than 250 days with those with earlier progression with a sensitivity of 75% and specificity of 100%. This was compared with RECIST 1.1, which had sensitivity and specificity of 16% and 100%, respectively, and modified Choi with 93% and 44%, respectively. However, the criteria required three-dimensional volumetric evaluation that required proprietary software, limiting adoption for clinical use.[1]

The Morphology, Attenuation, Size, and Structure criteria were developed to overcome limitations of the SACT criteria. It eliminated three-dimensional analysis and defined specific patterns that were based on changes in lesion morphology, attenuation, and size of target lesions in the portal venous phase of CT. This set of criteria separated response into favorable, indeterminate, and unfavorable categories. A major change from the others was that greater than or equal to 40% decrease in attenuation or marked necrosis was considered a favorable response.[28]

Given the development of antiangiogenic drugs that induce stabilization rather than tumor regression, criteria of RECIST 1.1 may be inadequate in early detection of progressive disease because it is based only on tumor size. Therefore, these alternate classifications that incorporate attenuation, morphology, and structural changes are likely to provide more accurate indication of response. However, there are limitations in reproducibility and the prognostic value of these imaging-based tumor response criteria may differ based on clinical risk status.[23] Therefore, it is yet to be determined how the changes in imaging appearance should guide the management of patients with metastatic RCC, to

Table 3
The development of various tumor response assessment systems reflects the advancement of pharmaceutical agents

System	Criteria/Target Lesions	Complete Response	Partial Response	Stable Disease	Progressive Disease
RECIST 1.1	Tumor size ≥10 mm Maximum of 5 target lesions (maximum 2 per organ)	Disappearance of all target lesions Any pathologic lymph nodes (TL or NTL) must have reduction in short axis to <10 mm	≥30% decrease in the sum of the longest dimensions of the target lesions, with the baseline sum of the diameters as reference	Does not qualify as partial disease or progressive disease	≥30% increase in the sum of the longest diameters of the target lesions, with the smallest sum as reference Sum must also have absolute increase of a minimum of 5 mm New lesions
Choi	Tumor size ≥15 mm Maximum of 10 target lesions Lesion attenuation as measured on portal venous phase	Disappearance of all lesions No new lesions	≥10% decrease in size (unidimensional in axial) OR a decrease in tumor attenuation of ≥15% HU No new lesions No obvious progression of measurable disease	Does not meet the criteria for CR, PR, or PD No symptomatic deterioration attributed to tumor progression	≥10% increase in tumor size (unidimensional in axial) and does not meet criteria of PR by tumor attenuation New lesions
Modified Choi	Tumor size ≥15 mm Maximum of 10 target lesions Lesion attenuation as measured on arterial phase	Disappearance of all lesions No new lesions	≥10% decrease in size (unidimensional in axial) AND a decrease in tumor attenuation of ≥15% HU No new lesions No obvious progression of measurable disease	Does not meet the criteria for CR, PR, or PD No symptomatic deterioration attributed to tumor progression	≥10% increase in tumor size (unidimensional in axial) and does not meet criteria of PR by tumor attenuation New lesions New intratumoral nodules or increase in the size of the existing intratumoral nodules

System	Criteria/Target Lesions	Favorable Response	Indeterminate Response	Unfavorable Response
SACT	Tumor size ≥10 mm Maximum of 10 target lesions (maximum 5 per organ) Patterns of contrast enhancement as determined on portal venous phase VOI Lung lesions are not measured using attenuation or volume	Decrease in tumor size VOI of 20% Decrease in tumor size (VOI) of ≥10% AND a. ≥20 HU decrease in mean attenuation of half or more of the nonlung target lesions ≥40 HU decreased mean attenuation of ≥1 nonlung target lesions	Does not fit criteria for favorable or unfavorable response	Increase in tumor size (VOI) of ≥20% New metastases Marked central fill-in New enhancement of a previously homogenous hypoattenuating nonenhancing mass
MASS	Tumor size ≥10 mm Maximum of 10 target lesions (maximum 5 per organ) Lesion attenuation as measured on portal venous phase Brain lesions excluded Lung lesions were not assessed for marked central necrosis or marked decreased attenuation	No new lesion AND a. Decrease in tumor size (longest axial dimension) of ≥20% ≥1 predominantly solid enhancing lesions with marked central necrosis or marked decreased attenuation (≥40 HU)	Does not fit criteria for favorable or unfavorable response	Increase in tumor size (longest axial dimension) of ≥20% New metastases Marked central fill-in New enhancement of a previously homogenous hypoattenuating nonenhancing mass

Several systems incorporate features other than lesion size, given the cytostatic nature of current first-line therapeutic agents.

Abbreviations: CR, complete response; NTL, non-target lesion; PD, progressive disease; PR, partial response; TL, target lesion; MASS, Morphology, Attenuation, Size, and Structure; RECIST 1.1, Response Evaluation Criteria in Solid Tumors 1.1; SACT, Size and Attenuation CT; VOI, volume of interest.

maximize cancer-specific outcomes.[1] Despite its shortcomings, RECIST 1.1 remains the widely accepted standardized method in most trials of solid tumors.[29]

OTHER IMAGING MODALITIES
Role of Ultrasound

Ultrasound is rarely used for staging evaluation of RCC. There are many challenges in ultrasound and image quality is user dependent. Challenges include incomplete visualization of masses, acoustic shadowing from partially calcified cysts or masses, variability in echogenicity of hemorrhagic cysts and malignant tumors, and poor sensitivity in diagnosing isoechoic small renal tumors. Hence, ultrasound seldom is used for local staging of RCC,[16] and when iodinated contrast used for CT is contraindicated, MRI is favorable as compared with ultrasound.

Role of Nuclear Medicine

The role of PET/CT staging and metastatic work-up in RCC is evolving.[16] PET/CT sequentially acquires PET images and a CT scan, usually in a single system where both scanners are fitted into a single gantry, which allows coregistered images of PET and CT scans to be provided.[16] FDG accumulation inside RCC cells depends on the expression of glucose transporter-1.[4] 18F-FDG-PET/CT is a useful adjunct to conventional imaging in establishing metastatic disease in lesions detected by CT, MRI, or bone scan. 18F-FDG-PET/CT is used in high-risk RCC patients with better sensitivity for detecting distant metastasis, providing anatomic and metabolic information.[4] However, the high background of renal pelvis from physiologic excretion of FDG limits evaluation of small primary RCC.[16] Although the usefulness of 18F-FDG-PET/CT in primary RCC remains unclear, and FDG-PET/CT is not currently recommended for the diagnosis and staging of RCC based on updated national and international guidelines.[4] Another PET agent, 18F-NaF, was Food and Drug Administration approved in 2016, and has been shown to be more sensitive in detecting bone metastasis with the greatest impact in initial staging and monitoring of bone lesions.[16]

99mTc-MDP bone scintigraphy is typically used for surveillance for skeletal metastases and is currently considered a sensitive but not specific tool for detecting metastatic bone lesions of RCC.[17] In a study of 124 patients with clinically localized, stages T1-2N0M0 disease, only six (5%) were found to have bone metastasis and it was therefore suggested that bone scans should be reserved for symptomatic patients who develop specific symptoms, such as local pain or abnormal alkaline phosphatase levels.[16]

Newer PET agents, such as prostate-specific membrane antigen (PSMA) targeting, are being researched to aid in detection of metastatic RCC. PSMA is a type II transmembrane protein with high expression in prostate carcinoma cells and has been suggested as a novel tracer that can detect prostate carcinoma relapses and metastases with high target-to-background ratio. PSMA-PET has shown promising results in clinical trials for detecting the recurrence of prostate cancer, although it is not yet Food and Drug Administration approved in the United States. In addition to prostate cancer, PSMA is expressed in the endothelial cells within the neovasculature of various solid malignant tumors including clear cell RCC.[30] In a case report by Demirci and colleagues[28] multiple pathologic bone lesions were found to have better visual detectability on 68-Ga-PSMA over FDG-PET.[30] Rowe and colleagues[31] reported five patients with metastatic RCC with more accurate staging for metastatic RCC. In all five patients, sites of metastatic disease were easily detectable through abnormal uptake of 18F-DCFPyL (inhibitor of PMSA), with more lesions detected than on conventional imaging. PET-detected sites included lymph nodes, pancreatic parenchymal lesions, lung parenchymal lesions, a brain parenchymal lesion, and other soft tissue sites. However, the subtype of RCC seems to play a role in PSMA receptor expressivity because PSMA-based PET (18F-DCFPyL) may show uptake infrequently in non–clear cell RCC. PSMA binds to endothelial cells within the tumor microenvironment. Therefore, it is proposed that higher pretreatment levels of radiotracer uptake may identify lesions that are more likely to respond to angiogenesis-targeted therapies and thereby aiding clinicians in treatment strategies.[31]

Another novel radiotracer, 124I-cG250, used in conjunction with PET/CT has been reported to assist in characterizing clear cell subtype RCC. G250 and its chimeric form cG250 (girentuximab) are monoclonal antibodies that recognize CAIX (carboxyl anhydrase IX transmembrane) on the cell membrane of clear cell RCC, and CAIX is known to be highly expressed in clear cell subtype RCC.[32] Two clinical trials by Divgi and colleagues[33,34] investigate this agent and have shown promising results in distinguishing clear subtype, but predominantly on larger masses, where the sensitivity was 89.4% in 2- to 4-cm tumors but only 70.8% in tumors less than 2 cm. The size limitation, in fact, may be driven by the [124]I PET imaging properties, such as long-range positron emission in tissue (3 mm) and emission of 50% of positrons simultaneously with high-energy (603 keV) photons, which leads to increase in background counts and degradation of image contrast. Thus, sensitivity and specificity for detecting small (<4 cm) clear cell RCC lesions is yet to be determined and more investigative work needs to be conducted in a larger study with histologic reference.[32]

SUMMARY

Because metastatic disease is common in RCC at initial presentation and even after surgical treatment, accurate staging evaluation is important for suitable treatment. In addition, assessment of response to therapy is an important indicator for change in the choice of systemic therapeutic agents. CT and MRI are the mainstay of imaging tests for metastatic RCC evaluation, with other modalities being used only for symptomatic patients. The complementary strengths of different imaging modalities may assist with determination of disease extent and treatment selection as application of the most sensitive imaging modality based on organs of concern can aid detection of metastatic disease. Understanding the accuracy of the available imaging options may in part mitigate against unnecessarily frequent screening for metastatic disease. For assessment of response to systemic therapy, evidence suggests that considering size and attenuation may provide more prognostic information but a single system for such evaluation is not yet widely established. As disease-specific outcomes of new chemotherapeutic agents become clearer, the data may guide more precise imaging assessment of tumor response. One imaging technique under active investigation is nuclear medicine, because newer agents, such as PMSA, show potential for improved detection of metastases and further studies are needed to establish clinical utility.

DISCLOSURE

Dr S.K. Kang reports royalties from Wolters Kluwer for unrelated work. Dr E. Zan is involved in clinical trial support at AAA/Novartis and Perlmutter Cancer Center for unrelated work, and acting as a Co-PI in a study at the NIH for unrelated work. Dr S.V.L. Vig has no disclosures.

REFERENCES

1. Nathan PD, Vinayan A, Stott D, Juttla J, Goh V. CT response assessment combining reduction in both size and arterial phase density correlates with time to progression in metastatic renal cancer patients treated with targeted therapies. Cancer Biol Ther 2010;9(1):15–9.

2. Janzen NK, Kim HL, Figlin RA, et al. Surveillance after radical or partial nephrectomy for localized renal cell carcinoma and management of recurrent disease. Urol Clin North Am 2003;30(4):843–52.

3. Griffin N, Gore ME, Sohaib SA. Imaging in metastatic renal cell carcinoma. AJR Am J Roentgenol 2007; 189(2):360–70.

4. Win AZ, Aparici CM. Clinical effectiveness of (18)F-fluorodeoxyglucose positron emission tomography/computed tomography in management of renal cell carcinoma: a single institution experience. World J Nucl Med 2015;14(1):36–40.

5. Diaz de Leon A, Pedrosa I. Imaging and screening of kidney cancer. Radiol Clin North Am 2017;55(6):1235–50.

6. Hutson TE, Thoreson GR, Figlin RA, et al. The Evolution of Systemic Therapy in Metastatic Renal Cell Carcinoma. Am Soc Clin Oncol Educ Book 2016; 35:113–7.

7. Coppin C, Porzsolt F, Awa A, et al. Immunotherapy for advanced renal cell cancer. Cochrane Database Syst Rev 2005;(1):CD001425.

8. Motzer RJ, Rini BI, Bukowski RM, et al. Sunitinib in patients with metastatic renal cell carcinoma. JAMA 2006;295(21):2516–24.

9. Weinstock M, McDermott D. Targeting PD-1/PD-L1 in the treatment of metastatic renal cell carcinoma. Ther Adv Urol 2015;7(6):365–77.

10. Motzer J, Thomas Powles, Michael B. Atkins, et al. IMmotion151: a randomized phase III study of atezolizumab plus bevacizumab vs sunitinib in untreated metastatic renal cell carcinoma (mRCC). Journal of Clinical Oncology, 2018;36(6_suppl):578.

11. Ng CS, Wood CG, Silverman PM, et al. Renal cell carcinoma: diagnosis, staging, and surveillance. AJR Am J Roentgenol 2008;191(4):1220–32.

12. Patel U, Sokhi H. Imaging in the follow-up of renal cell carcinoma. AJR Am J Roentgenol 2012;198(6):1266–76.

13. Wu Y, Kwon YS, Labib M, et al. Magnetic resonance imaging as a biomarker for renal cell carcinoma. Dis Markers 2015;2015:648495.

14. Ljungberg B, LA, Bensalah K, et al. EAU oncology guidelines for renal cell carcinoma. Eur Assoc Urol 2019;75(5):799–810.

15. Campbell S, Uzzo RG, Allaf ME, et al. Renal mass and localized renal cancer: AUA guideline. J Urol 2017;198(3):520–9.

16. Vikram R, Beland MD, Blaufox MD, et al. ACR Appropriateness Criteria Renal Cell Carcinoma Staging. J Am Coll Radiol 2016;13(5):518–25.

17. Koga S, Tsuda S, Nishikido M, et al. The diagnostic value of bone scan in patients with renal cell carcinoma. J Urol 2001;166(6):2126–8.

18. Bachor R, Kotzerke J, Gottfried HW, et al. [Positron emission tomography in diagnosis of renal cell carcinoma]. Urologe A 1996;35(2):146–50.

19. Kang DE, White RL Jr, Zuger JH, et al. Clinical use of fluorodeoxyglucose F 18 positron emission tomography for detection of renal cell carcinoma. J Urol 2004;171(5):1806–9.

20. Lordan JT, Fawcett WJ, Karanjia ND. Solitary liver metastasis of chromophobe renal cell carcinoma 20 years after nephrectomy treated by hepatic resection. Urology 2008;72(1):230.e5-6.

21. Koneru R, Hotte SJ. Role of cytokine therapy for renal cell carcinoma in the era of targeted agents. Curr Oncol 2009;16(Suppl 1):S40–4.

22. Krajewski KM, Nishino M, Ramaiya NH, et al. RECIST 1.1 compared with RECIST 1.0 in patients with advanced renal cell carcinoma receiving vascular endothelial growth factor-targeted therapy. AJR Am J Roentgenol 2015;204(3):W282–8.

23. Kang HC, Gupta S, Wei W, et al. Alternative Response Criteria and Clinical Risk Factors for Assessing Tumor Response in Patients With Metastatic Renal Cell Carcinoma Who Are Receiving Salvage Therapy. AJR Am J Roentgenol. 2017;209(6):1278–84.

24. Joern Henze DM. Thorsten Persigehl, RECIST 1.1, ir-RECIST 1.1, and mRECIST: how to do. Curr Radiol Rep 2016;4:1–11.

25. Choi H. Response evaluation of gastrointestinal stromal tumors. Oncologist 2008;13(suppl 2):4–7.

26. Van der Veldt AA, Meijerink MR, van den Eertwegh AJ, Haanen JB, Boven E. Choi response criteria for early prediction of clinical outcome in patients with metastatic renal cell cancer treated with sunitinib. Br J Cancer 2010;102(5):803–9.

27. Smith AD, Lieber ML, Shah SN. Assessing tumor response and detecting recurrence in metastatic renal cell carcinoma on targeted therapy: importance of size and attenuation on contrast-enhanced CT. AJR Am J Roentgenol 2010;194(1):157–65.

28. Demirci E, Ocak M, Kabasakal L, et al. ^{68}Ga-PSMA PET/CT imaging of metastatic clear cell renal cell carcinoma. Eur J Nucl Med Mol Imaging 2014;41:1461–2.

29. Schwartz LH, Litiere S, de Vries E, et al. RECIST 1.1-Update and clarification: From the RECIST committee. Eur J Cancer 2016;62:132–7.

30. Baccala A, Sercia L, Li J, et al. Expression of prostate-specific membrane antigen in tumor-associated neovasculature of renal neoplasms. Urology 2007;70(2):385–90.

31. Rowe SP, Gorin MA, Hammers HJ, et al. Imaging of metastatic clear cell renal cell carcinoma with PSMA-targeted (1)(8)F-DCFPyL PET/CT. Annals of nuclear medicine 2015;29(10):877–82.

32. Khandani AH, Rathmell WK, Wallen EM, et al. PET/CT with (124)I-cG250: great potential and some open questions. AJR Am J Roentgenol 2014;203(2):261–2.

33. Divgi CR, Pandit-Taskar N, Jungbluth AA, et al. Pre-operative characterisation of clear-cell renal carcinoma using iodine-124-labelled antibody chimeric G250 (124I-cG250) and PET in patients with renal masses: a phase I trial. Lancet Oncol 2007;8(4):304–10.

34. Divgi CR, Uzzo RG, Gatsonis C, et al. Positron emission tomography/computed tomography identification of clear cell renal cell carcinoma: results from the REDECT trial. J Clin Oncol 2013;31(2):187–94.

Epidemiology, Risk Assessment, and Biomarkers for Patients with Advanced Renal Cell Carcinoma

Kyrollis Attalla, MD, Stanley Weng, MS, Martin H. Voss, MD, A Ari Hakimi, MD*

KEYWORDS

- Immunotherapy • Metastatic renal cell carcinoma • Predictive biomarker • Prognostic biomarker
- Risk assessment • Targeted therapy

KEY POINTS

- Renal cell carcinoma (RCC) is the most lethal urologic malignancy and is the eighth leading cause of cancer in the United States, comprising 3% of adult malignancies. The 5-year survival of patients with metastatic disease is approximately 12%.
- Distinct clinical variables were found to associate with prognosis, and identifying patients likely to derive benefit from specific therapies or cytoreductive strategies posed a significant clinical challenge.
- Prognostic models were developed from these identified clinical factors that were predicated upon disease burden, tumor, and patient-related factors. The most widely used models include the Memorial Sloan Kettering Cancer Center risk model and the International Metastatic RCC Database Consortium model.
- Biomarker development in metastatic RCC is an emerging field of research; the most widely studied biomarkers include prognostic models as predictive biomarkers, genomic and gene-expression based biomarkers, and molecular and immunohistochemical biomarkers.
- Advances in prognostication and biomarker development will be aided by further insight into the biological processes underlying the development of metastatic RCC and the development of powerful biomarkers validated for use in routine clinical practice.

INTRODUCTION

Renal cell carcinoma (RCC) accounts for 3% of adult malignancies and is the eighth leading cause of cancer in the United States.[1] Worldwide, 400,000 people were diagnosed and 175,000 people died of kidney cancer in 2018. Up to 30% of patients diagnosed with RCC present with synchronous metastases, and recurrence is seen in 30% of patients after complete resection of the primary tumor.[2,3] Although the 5-year survival of early-stage RCC is 93%, patients presenting with metastatic disease have dismal 5-year survival rates of approximately 12%, and at least half of patients with RCC will eventually require systemic therapy.[4] RCC is generally considered resistant to conventional cytotoxic chemotherapy and radiotherapy but has classically been regarded as an immunogenic tumor as evidenced by occasional spontaneous regressions and mild to moderate success with prior immunotherapeutic approaches.[5]

Department of Surgery, Urology Service, Memorial Sloan Kettering Cancer Center, 353 East 68th Street, 5th Floor, New York, NY 10065, USA
* Corresponding author.
E-mail address: hakimia@mskcc.org

Urol Clin N Am 47 (2020) 293–303
https://doi.org/10.1016/j.ucl.2020.04.002
0094-0143/20/© 2020 Elsevier Inc. All rights reserved.

Before 2005, the only approved treatment of metastatic renal cell carcinoma (mRCC) was high-dose interleukin-2, which exhibited durable responses in approximately 5% to 10% of patients at the cost of severe acute toxicities as a result of the proinflammatory cytokine storm induced by treatment.[6] Low-dose subcutaneous interferon (IFN) was commonly used instead, given its somewhat better safety profile, although durable responses were uncommon. After 2005, the treatment landscape for mRCC shifted from immunotherapeutic approaches to approaches directed at growth factors overexpressed in RCC downstream of altered von Hippel–Lindau (VHL) function, particularly vascular endothelial growth factor (VEGF). Several multitargeted tyrosine kinase inhibitors with activity against the VEGF receptor, antibodies directed against VEGF, and small molecule inhibitors of mammalian target of rapamycin were explored in mRCC leading to Food and Drug Administration approval and integration as standard therapies. Despite the plethora of such therapies introduced to treat mRCC, and the convenience of oral administration offered by many of these drugs, chronic administration is required, adverse effects can substantially impact quality of life, and the vast majority of patients ultimately experience disease progression despite treatment.[7]

In just a few years since entering the clinic, immune checkpoint blockade (ICB) has dramatically changed the landscape of treatment of mRCC and has secured a place as a standard pillar of treatment. Despite these successes and a renewed enthusiasm for immunotherapy, mRCC still carries a poor prognosis and remains unpredictable with a highly variable clinical course, spanning from indolent to rapidly progressing disease. Because distinct clinical variables were found to associate with prognosis, identifying patients likely to derive benefit from specific therapies or cytoreductive strategies posed a significant clinical challenge. Indeed, prognostic models were developed from these identified clinical factors, which were predicated upon disease burden, tumor, and patient-related factors. In this review, we outline investigated biomarkers and the risk assessment tools developed to better inform therapeutic decisions and accurately prognosticate patients with mRCC.

RISK-STRATIFICATION MODELS

Prognostic models are critical components of clinical trial design, risk-directed therapy, and patient counseling. Prognostic factors differ from predictive factors in that prognostic factors associate with progression and survival of patients, whereas predictive factors refer to the effects of therapeutic agents to

the tumor or host.[8] An observation first noted during the cytokine era, prognosis in mRCC varies with the involved target organ with liver and bone involvement portending worse survival compared with lung and regional lymph node metastasis.[9]

One of the first and most widely used prognostic models, the Memorial Sloan Kettering Cancer Center (MSKCC) model, reported by Motzer and colleagues[10,11] used pooled data from patients in clinical trials treated with IFN-alpha accrued from 1982 to 1996 to identify 5 prognostic factors. These factors included Karnofsky performance status (KPS; <80%), serum lactate dehydrogenase (LDH; >1.5× upper limit of normal [ULN]), hemoglobin level (< lower limit of normal), level of corrected serum calcium (>10 mg/dL), and time from initial RCC diagnosis to start of therapy of less than 1 year. Using this model, patients stratified in the favorable-risk group have zero factors (median overall survival [OS], 29.6 months); patients stratified in the intermediate-risk group have one or 2 risk factors (median OS, 13.8 months), and patients stratified in the poor-risk group have 3 or more risk factors (median OS, 4.9 months). In a validation study, Mekhail and colleagues[12] added prior radiotherapy and number of metastatic sites the MSKCC model, terming this extended model the Cleveland Clinic Foundation (CCF) model.

The shift from the cytokine era to the targeted therapy era was accompanied by a need for updated prognostic models and survival estimates. Using a cohort of 645 patients with mRCC treated with sunitinib, sorafenib, and IFN-alpha plus bevacizumab, Heng and colleagues[13] developed a new prognostic model termed the International mRCC Database Consortium (IMDC) model. Four of the 5 MSKCC criteria were found to be prognostic; LDH was not significantly associated with survival in this model. Two additional factors, neutrophilia (> ULN) and thrombocythemia (> ULN), were independently associated with survival. The IMDC model was externally validated in a cohort of patients treated with first-line VEGF-targeted therapy and compared with other prognostic models, including MSKCC, CCF, the International Kidney Cancer Working Group (IKCWG), and Groupe Francais d'Immunotherapie.[14] Patients in the favorable-risk group have zero factors with a median OS that was not reached (43.2 months in the external validation cohort); patients in the intermediate-risk group have one or 2 risk factors (median OS, 27 months), and patients in the poor-risk group have 3 or more risk factors (median OS, 8.8 months).

Over a period of 6 years, the Groupe Français d'Immunothérapie enrolled 782 mRCC patients treated with cytokine regimens to identify prognostic factors for survival, demonstrating that performance status, number of metastatic sites, disease-free interval, biological signs of inflammation, and hemoglobin levels can be considered validated prognostic factors.[15] Four independent factors predictive of rapid progression in patients treated with cytokine therapy were likewise identified, including the presence of hepatic metastases, short interval from renal tumor to metastases (<1 year), more than 1 metastatic site, and elevated neutrophil counts. Patients with at least 3 of these factors have greater than 80% probability of rapid progression despite treatment.

The IKCWG model used a database of 3748 patients pooled from clinical trials and was validated using an independent data set of 645 patients treated with tyrosine kinase inhibitors.[16] Nine clinical factors were identified as prognostic, including prior treatment, performance status, number of metastatic sites, time from diagnosis to treatment, pretreatment hemoglobin, white blood cell count, LDH, alkaline phosphatase, and serum calcium. Three risk groups were formed: favorable, intermediate-risk, and poor-risk groups with a median survival of 26.9 months, 11.5 months, and 4.2 months, respectively. **Table 1** compares clinical factors across models, and **Table 2** demonstrates the risk-stratification and survival estimates of the available prognostic models in mRCC.

The clinical course of patients with mRCC spans a wide spectrum, and distinct factors appear to forecast a more aggressive course of disease. RCC frequently metastasizes to the lung (60%–70%), regional lymph nodes (60%–65%), bone (39%–40%), liver (19%–40%), and brain (5%–7%).[17] Vickers and colleagues[18] examined 15% of patients with mRCC and brain metastases from the IMDC to demonstrate that OS was worse in patients with more than 4 brain metastases, compared with those with less than 4 metastases (3.9 vs 15.4 months, $P = .005$) McKay and colleagues[19] similarly used the IMDC to analyze outcomes based on the presence of bone and liver metastases in patients treated with targeted therapy. Bone metastases were present in 34% of the 2027 patients in the consortium and were present in all risk groups but highest in poor-risk patients (43%, $P<.001$). Median OS was worse in patients with bone metastases compared with those without (14.9 vs 25.1 months, $P = .0001$). Similarly, liver metastases accounted for 19% of the group, were highest in poor-risk patients (23%, $P = .003$), and demonstrated worse median OS compared with those without liver metastases (14.3 vs 22.2 months, $P<.001$).

Risk Stratification in the Second-Line Setting

The development of risk-stratification models in the second-line setting was largely hampered by

---

Table 1
Prognostic models in advanced renal cell carcinoma

Prognostic Factors	MSKCC Motzer et al,[11] 2002	IMDC Heng et al,[13] 2009	GFI Negrier et al,[15] 2002	CCF Mekhail et al,[12] 2005	IKCWG Manola et al,[16] 2011
Performance status	●	●	●		●
Elevated serum LDH	●			●	●
Low hemoglobin	●	●	●	●	●
High corrected serum Ca	●	●		●	●
Time from Dx to Tx <1 y	●	●	● ○	●	●
Prior radiotherapy				●	
Number of metastatic sites			● ○	●	●
Hepatic metastasis			○		
Elevated ANC		●	○		● (WBC)
Elevated platelets		●			
Inflammation			●		
Elevated ALP					●
Prior immunotherapy					●

Abbreviations: ●, prognostic factors for survival; ○, prognostic factors for rapid progression; ALP, alkaline phosphatase; ANC, absolute neutrophil count; Dx, diagnosis; GFI, Groupe Français d'Immunothérapie; Tx, therapy; WBC, white blood cells.

Table 2
Risk categorization of prognostic models in advanced renal cell carcinoma

Risk Category	MSKCC	Median Survival, mo	IMDC	Median Survival, mo	GFI	Median Survival, mo	CCF	Median Survival, mo	IKCWG	Median Survival, mo
Good/ favorable	0	30	0	43	0–1	42	0	26	RS[a] < −2.76	26.9
Intermediate	1–2	14	1–2	22.5	2–3	15	1	14.4	−2.76 < RS ≤ −1.25	11.6
Poor	≥3	5	≥3	7.8	4–5	6	≥3	7.3	RS ≥ −1.25	4.2

Abbreviation: RS, risk score.
[a] Cutoff points for risk scores are placed at the 25th and 75th percentiles of the models' risk score distribution as per Manola and colleagues.[16]

the poor survival seen in patients with mRCC in the cytokine era. As targeted therapy began to supplant traditional immunotherapy in the treatment of patients with mRCC, survival improved from less than 1 year in the cytokine era to approximately 24 months with targeted therapy.[20,21] Motzer and colleagues[22] pooled 251 patients from 29 clinical trials between 1975 and 2002 to describe the survival of patients who were candidates for second-line therapy with novel agents after progression on cytokine therapy. Pretreatment features associated with shorter survival appeared to be low KPS, low hemoglobin level, and high corrected serum calcium. By use of these risk factors, patients were categorized into 3 groups: patients with zero risk factors (median OS, 22 months); patients with 1 risk factor (median OS, 11.9 months); and patients with 2 to 3 risk factors (median OS, 5.4 months). Subsequently, in 2015, Ko and colleagues[23] sought to validate the IMDC model in patients with mRCC receiving next-line targeted therapy after progression on first-line targeted therapy. In a cohort of 1021 patients who received second-line targeted therapy, median OS since the start of second-line therapy was 12.5 months, and when compared with the MSKCC model, the IMDC model conferred a better concordance index (0.70 vs 0.66). Using the 3 risk categories per IMDC criteria, median OS was 35.3 months in favorable-risk patients, 16.6 months in intermediate-risk patients, and 5.4 months in poor-risk patients.

Non–Clear Cell Metastatic Renal Cell Carcinoma

The predominant histologic subtype of RCC is clear cell RCC, which accounts for 70% to 80% of all kidney cancers. Data collected from the IMDC demonstrated the median OS of patients with non–clear cell mRCC treated with novel targeted agents to be significantly poorer than patients with clear cell RCC (12.8 vs 22.3 months, $P<.0001$).[24] The prognosis of patients with papillary RCC is significantly worse than their clear cell and chromophobe counterparts, and similarly, sarcomatoid RCC was found to carry an even poorer prognosis, with the percentage of sarcomatoid component potentially inferring worse OS.[24–26] A report from the IMDC by Kyriakopoulos and colleagues[27] showed patients with sarcomatoid histology have a shorter time to relapse, worse baseline prognostic criteria, and worse clinical outcome with targeted therapy with a progression-free survival (PFS) and median OS of 4.5 and 10.4 months, respectively. The aforementioned prognostic models in mRCC, however, were developed based on clinical and laboratory values, without consideration of histologic subtype. Given the worse clinical behavior of non–clear cell RCCs, Kroeger and colleagues[24] aimed to characterize the applicability of the IMDC prognostic model to non–clear cell subtypes. The same IMDC criteria and risk categories still reliably predicted time to treatment failure and OS in this cohort of patients; the median OS of favorable-, intermediate-, and poor-prognosis groups were 31.4, 16.1, and 5.1 months, respectively.

BIOMARKERS IN ADVANCED RENAL CELL CARCINOMA

As the era of precision oncology dawns, significant challenges lie in identifying biomarkers applicable in both clinical and research settings. Biomarkers are objective, quantifiable characteristics of biological processes. When used as outcomes in clinical trials, biomarkers are considered to be surrogate endpoints; however, sound scientific evidence that a biomarker consistently and accurately predicts a clinical outcome must exist. In such context, a surrogate endpoint is a biomarker that can be trusted to serve as a stand-in for, but not as a replacement of, a clinical endpoint.[28] Stated differently, biomarkers may effectively be used as true replacements for clinically relevant endpoints if the normal physiology and pathophysiology of a biological process and the effects of interventions are completely understood; because this is rarely the case, the relevance and validity of biomarkers require iterative reassessment.

Risk Models as a Predictive Biomarker

Currently, biomarker development in mRCC is an emerging and evolving field of research because biomarkers are integral in delivering risk-directed therapies. Many of the clinical variables comprising the above risk-stratification models are potential biomarkers predictive of outcome because they are objective and quantifiable. To date, the only predictive biomarker prospectively validated in a phase 3 randomized controlled trial is the IMDC risk model, which was later validated in several other mRCC subsets, including non–clear cell RCC, in the second-, third-, and fourth-line settings, and in patients treated with ICB.[29] Data from Checkmate 214, a phase 3 trial comparing nivolumab plus ipilimumab versus sunitinib for previously untreated advanced clear-cell RCC, demonstrated patients with intermediate- or poor-risk disease had favorable clinical outcomes with combination ICB versus sunitinib.[30]

Genomic Biomarkers

Risk-stratification models leverage clinical and biochemical parameters to prognosticate patients; however, increasingly sophisticated molecular characterizations make it likely that genomic parameters will also be used in the prognostication of patients with mRCC. Large-scale sequencing efforts have helped characterize the genomic landscape of clear cell RCC.[31,32] VHL, a tumor suppressor gene located on chromosome 3p25, is the most commonly mutated gene in clear cell RCC and is involved in the regulation of hypoxia-inducible factor-α and angiogenesis.[32] Three additional tumor suppressor genes, PBRM1, SETD2, and BAP1, are located on the same 3p chromosomal region, and after VHL, comprise the most commonly mutated genes in clear cell RCC.[31] Until recently, scant data existed regarding the correlation between genomic alterations and outcomes in patients with metastatic RCC; Carlo and

colleagues[33] explored the relationship between mutational profile and cancer-specific outcomes in a review of 105 patients with metastatic clear cell RCC who received prior VEGF-targeted therapy. The presence of BAP1 or TERT mutations was associated with significantly worse OS, whereas mutations in PBRM1 seemed to correlate with longer time to treatment failure and a trend toward superior OS.

In an effort to determine if the addition of the mutation status for several candidate prognostic genes to the MSKCC model could improve the model's prognostic performance, Voss and colleagues[34] leveraged 2 independent clinical trial datasets (COMPARZ trial [training cohort; n = 357] and RECORD-3 trial [validation cohort; n = 258]) of patients with mRCC treated with first-line targeted therapies. In the training cohort, the presence of any mutation in BAP1 or TP53, or both, was associated with inferior OS (hazard ratio [HR] = 1.58; P = .0008) as well as absence of any mutation in PBRM1 (HR = 1.58; P = .0035). The mutation status for these 3 prognostic genes was then added to the original MSKCC risk model to create a genomically annotated version. Addition of genomic information improved model performance for predicting OS (c-index: original model, 0.595 vs new model, 0.637) and PFS (0.567 vs 0.602), and analyses in the validation cohort confirmed the superiority of the genomically annotated risk model over the original version. Similar efforts by Hsieh and colleagues[35] aimed to evaluate the relationship between tumor mutations and treatment outcomes in RECORD-3. Among the cohort, prevalent somatic mutations were VHL (75%), PBRM1 (46%), SETD2 (30%), BAP1 (19%), KDM5C (15%), and PTEN (12%). With first-line everolimus, PBRM1 and BAP1 mutations were associated with longer (12.8 vs 5.5 months) and shorter (4.9 vs 10.5 months) median first-line PFS, and with first-line sunitinib, KDM5C mutations were associated with longer median first-line PFS (20.6 vs 8.3 months), providing compelling evidence that molecular subgroups of metastatic clear cell RCC based on the somatic mutations they harbor could have predictive values for patients treated with targeted therapy.

Recent work from several groups pointed to the association of immunotherapy response and mutations in the SWI/SNF chromatin remodeling complex, more specifically the polybromo and BRG-1 associated factors (PBAF) complex, which include the genes ARID2, PBRM1, and BRD7.[36–38] Miao and colleagues[36] demonstrated that in a series of nearly 100 metastatic clear cell RCC patients, those harboring loss-of-function mutations in PBRM1 had clinical benefit from ICB. Similarly, a recent report validated the association between *PBRM1* alterations and ICB response[39] in Check-Mate 025, a randomized phase 3 trial of nivolumab versus everolimus that demonstrated a survival benefit for nivolumab in the second- and third-line setting.[40] Further functional and transcriptomic analysis suggested that *PBRM1*-deficient tumors possessed altered immune signaling pathways. However, in IMmotion150, a phase 2 trial that randomized patients to first-line therapy with the anti–programmed death-ligand 1 (PD-L1) atezolizumab alone or combined to bevacizumab versus sunitinib, no association was seen between presence of *PBRM1* mutations and treatment response to the PD-L1–directed atezolizumab, nor to the combination of atezolizumab plus bevacizumab (n = 136); there was a favorable effect on treatment response in patients receiving sunitinib (anti-VEGF) on the control arm of the same study (n = 72).[41] Given the discordant clinical data on PBAF complex loss and response to immunotherapy, further investigation into its use as a biomarker is warranted.

Gene Expression Signatures

Several molecular gene signatures have been postulated and investigated as predictive of the efficacy of targeted therapy and immunotherapy. Beuselinck and colleagues[42] performed global transcriptome analyses on 53 primary resected clear cell RCC tumors from patients who developed metastatic disease treated with first-line sunitinib and identified 4 discrete molecular subtypes of clear cell RCC that were associated with outcome and response to sunitinib (ccrcc 1–4). The ccrcc2 (53%) and ccrcc3 (70%) subtypes were enriched in patients responding to sunitinib compared with ccrcc1 (22%) and ccrcc4 (27%), and ccrcc1 and ccrcc4 tumors had significantly shorter PFS and OS compared with the ccrcc2 and ccrcc3 subtypes. Similarly, recent data demonstrate that these molecular subtypes correlate well with IMDC risk groups.[42] Most good-risk patients (77%) had ccrcc2 tumors, which display a proangiogenic signature, whereas the ccrcc1 and ccrcc4 subtypes were almost exclusively found in intermediate- or poor-risk patients. These findings may explain the increased benefit of sunitinib over combined checkpoint blockade in good-risk patients in Checkmate 214.

A correlative study including 823 patients from IMmotion 151 demonstrated patients with tumors characterized by angiogenesis-high signatures experienced longer PFS with sunitinib when compared with those with angiogenesis-low tumors.[43] In addition, tumors with T-effector/IFN-γ-high or angiogenesis-low gene signatures displayed favorable outcomes with combination therapy compared with sunitinib. MSKCC favorable-risk patients were noted to be enriched with angiogenesis-high signatures, akin to the biologic rationale of the aforementioned CheckMate 214 trial, which suggested a greater dependency on angiogenic pathways in favorable-risk disease.

Key genomic and transcriptional determinants of response to tyrosine kinase inhibitors were derived by Hakimi and colleagues[44,45] from molecular features of archival tumor specimens collected in patients receiving pazopanib versus sunitinib in the phase 3 COMPARZ trial. Clustering of the expression microarray data identified 4 biologically distinct clusters that were associated with significant differences in median OS and response to tyrosine kinase inhibitors. Detailed characterization of these clusters emphasized the central role of the tumor microenvironment (TME) and identified angiogenesis and macrophage infiltration as critical determinants of response to therapy. Superior outcomes for patients with higher angiogenesis scores were noted, independent of IMDC risk category (HR for PFS and OS 0.68 and 0.68, respectively). The investigators postulate that upregulation and suppression of angiogenesis observed with loss-of-function mutations in *PBRM1* and *BAP1*, respectively, provide a plausible explanation for the different clinical behaviors associated with these mutations.

Programmed Death-Ligand 1 Immunohistochemical Expression

The first and most widely studied potential biomarker for response to anti–programmed cell death 1/PD-L1 agents is the immunohistochemical expression of PD-L1. CheckMate 025 demonstrated PD-L1 staining to be associated with worse survival but not associated with response to nivolumab, suggesting PD-L1 staining has more prognostic than predictive value in mRCC.[5] In both arms of the trial, an inferior OS was observed in patients with PD-L1 expression ≥1% compared with those with PD-L1 expression less than 1%. Nivolumab demonstrated a survival benefit over everolimus in both PD-L1 subgroups (median OS 21.8 vs 18.8 months in PD-L1 ≥1%, and 27.4 vs 21.2 months in PD-L1 <1%, respectively). Further supporting the notion of PD-L1 as a prognostic biomarker, Flaifel and colleagues[46] combined tumor tissue from 2 clinical trials, METEOR[47] (n = 306) and CABOSUN[48] (n = 110), showing higher PD-L1 expression resulted in worse clinical outcomes in mRCC treated with targeted therapy. In addition, PD-L1 expression was not predictive of response to cabozantinib.

With regard to response to ICB, exploratory analyses of intermediate- and poor-risk patients in CheckMate 214 demonstrated OS was 86% versus 66% at 12 months and 81% versus 53% at 18 months, favoring combination ICB over sunitinib, with median survival not reached versus 19.6 months (HR = 0.45, 95% confidence interval = 0.29–0.71) among patients with PD-L1 expression ≥1%.[30] Similarly, PD-L1 expression appeared to associate with improved overall response rate (ORR; 58% vs 22%) and median PFS (22.8 vs 5.9 months) in patients receiving combination ICB. Subsequently, in JAVELIN Renal 101, a phase 3 trial comparing avelumab plus axitinib with sunitinib in previously untreated patients with advanced RCC, the ORR among patients who received avelumab plus axitinib was double that among patients who received sunitinib, both among the patients with PD-L1–positive tumors and in the overall population (55.2% vs 25.5% and 51.4% vs 25.7%, respectively).[49] Similarly, among patients with PD-L1–positive tumors,

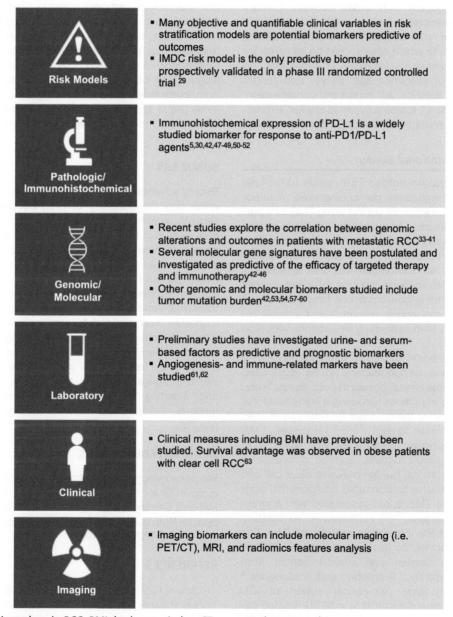

Risk Models
- Many objective and quantifiable clinical variables in risk stratification models are potential biomarkers predictive of outcomes
- IMDC risk model is the only predictive biomarker prospectively validated in a phase III randomized controlled trial [29]

Pathologic/ Immunohistochemical
- Immunohistochemical expression of PD-L1 is a widely studied biomarker for response to anti-PD1/PD-L1 agents[5,30,42,47-49,50-52]

Genomic/ Molecular
- Recent studies explore the correlation between genomic alterations and outcomes in patients with metastatic RCC[33-41]
- Several molecular gene signatures have been postulated and investigated as predictive of the efficacy of targeted therapy and immunotherapy[42-46]
- Other genomic and molecular biomarkers studied include tumor mutation burden[42,53,54,57-60]

Laboratory
- Preliminary studies have investigated urine- and serum-based factors as predictive and prognostic biomarkers
- Angiogenesis- and immune-related markers have been studied[61,62]

Clinical
- Clinical measures including BMI have previously been studied. Survival advantage was observed in obese patients with clear cell RCC[63]

Imaging
- Imaging biomarkers can include molecular imaging (i.e. PET/CT), MRI, and radiomics features analysis

Fig. 1. Biomarkers in RCC. BMI, body mass index; CT, computed tomography.

median PFS was significantly longer among patients who received avelumab plus axitinib than among those who received sunitinib (13.8 vs 7.2 months, $P<.001$). The IMmotion150 trial demonstrated a consistent trend of increasing efficacy with increasing levels of PD-L1, a finding further supported in the phase 3 study IMmotion151.[41,50] Finally, in KEYNOTE 426, the benefit of pembrolizumab plus axitinib over sunitinib with regards to OS and PFS was observed regardless of PD-L1 expression.[51]

In sum, PD-L1 expression has proven to be an inconsistent biomarker in RCC. The optimal threshold for PD-L1 positivity is ill defined, and the heterogeneity that exists between primary (including tumoral vs tumoral and immune infiltrate expression) and metastatic sites lends clinical dilemma as to which sites should be sampled for PD-L1 expression. Variability in expression on the basis of specimen age, assay, and vendor choice is likewise an important consideration. Because PD-L1 is also a dynamic marker, expression may be altered on the basis of prior therapy.

Tumor Mutational Burden

Tumor mutational burden (TMB) refers to the total number of mutations per coding area of tumor genome. The rationale behind using TMB as a predictive biomarker of response to ICB is that a higher mutational load may be accompanied by increased production of neoantigens, thereby stimulating an antitumoral immune response.[52] Prior studies in large cohorts of other cancer types, including non–small cell lung cancer and metastatic melanoma, demonstrate favorable responses to immunotherapy in patients with high TMB.[53–55]

Evidence from Checkmate 025 and Checkmate 214 showing immunotherapy to be associated with favorable clinical benefit in poor-risk patients, a subgroup of patients harboring a high mutational load, supported the rationale for research of TMB as a biomarker in RCC.[53,56,57] However, TMB does not appear to correlate with MSKCC or IMDC prognostic criteria, and no difference is seen in mutational burden between clear cell and more aggressive sarcomatoid components, suggesting that TMB is not associated with aggressivity of disease.[56,58] Furthermore, exploratory analysis of the previously mentioned IMmotion 150 trial showed no association between TMB or neoantigen burden and clinical benefit from ICB.[41] Recently, Samstein and colleagues[59] analyzed a large pan-cancer cohort of ICB (n = 1662) versus non-ICB (n = 5371) -treated patients whose tumors underwent targeted next-

generation sequencing. For most histologies, an association between higher TMB and improved survival was observed; however, the same association was not seen in RCC.

Several parameters spanning a wide spectrum of radiologic, pathologic, molecular, genomic, urine-, and serum-based factors have been investigated as predictive and prognostic biomarkers, although their study remains preliminary and not validated. A brief summary of biomarkers in RCC is outlined in **Fig. 1**. Angiogenesis-related parameters detected in blood are attractive as blood biomarkers because they are not subjected to tumor heterogeneity and allow longitudinal follow-up.[60] Immune-related adverse events have been explored as surrogate markers of pharmacodynamic effect, suggesting that mechanism-based toxicities may potentially serve as biomarkers.[61] Interestingly, a recent study by Sanchez and colleagues[62] found aspects of the TME that vary by body mass index in the tumor and peritumoral adipose tissue, possibly contributing to the observed survival advantage in obese patients with clear cell RCC.

SUMMARY

Recent advances in mRCC have shown promise in enhancing the accuracy of prognosticating patients through the integration of clinical, molecular, and genomic factors. As drug and biomarker development in mRCC continues to evolve, there yet remains an urgent need to improve patient selection for risk-directed treatment in the context of novel therapies, maximize the outcomes of these therapies, and minimize treatment-associated morbidity. Fundamental to accomplishing these efforts is further insight into the biological processes underlying the development of mRCC, the continual refinement of the discriminatory power of prognostic models, and the development and exacting reassessment of powerful biomarkers validated for use in routine clinical practice.

ACKNOWLEDEGEMENTS

We acknowledge support from the Cancer Center Support Grant of the National Institutes of Health/ National Cancer Institute (grant No P30CA008748) and the Ruth L. Kirschstein National Research Service Award T32CA082088.

REFERENCES

1. Bray F, Ferlay J, Soerjomataram I, et al. Global cancer statistics 2018: GLOBOCAN estimates of incidence and mortality worldwide for 36 cancers in

185 countries. CA Cancer J Clin 2018;68(6): 394–424.

2. Cohen HT, McGovern FJ. Renal-cell carcinoma. N Engl J Med 2005;353(23):2477–90.

3. Motzer RJ, Russo P, Nanus DM, et al. Renal cell carcinoma. Curr Probl Cancer 1997;21(4):185–232.

4. Siegel RL, Miller KD, Jemal A. Cancer statistics, 2017. CA Cancer J Clin 2017;67(1):7–30.

5. Itsumi M, Tatsugami K. Immunotherapy for renal cell carcinoma. Clin Dev Immunol 2010;2010:284581.

6. Fyfe G, Fisher RI, Rosenberg SA, et al. Results of treatment of 255 patients with metastatic renal cell carcinoma who received high-dose recombinant interleukin-2 therapy. J Clin Oncol 1995;13(3): 688–96.

7. Vaishampayan U, Vankayala H, Vigneau FD, et al. The effect of targeted therapy on overall survival in advanced renal cancer: a study of the National Surveillance Epidemiology and End Results registry database. Clin Genitourin Cancer 2014;12(2):124–9.

8. Sun M, Shariat SF, Cheng C, et al. Prognostic factors and predictive models in renal cell carcinoma: a contemporary review. Eur Urol 2011;60(4):644–61.

9. Naito S, Yamamoto N, Takayama T, et al. Prognosis of Japanese metastatic renal cell carcinoma patients in the cytokine era: a cooperative group report of 1463 patients. Eur Urol 2010;57(2):317–25.

10. Motzer RJ, Mazumdar M, Bacik J, et al. Survival and prognostic stratification of 670 patients with advanced renal cell carcinoma. J Clin Oncol 1999; 17(8):2530–40.

11. Motzer RJ, Bacik J, Murphy BA, et al. Interferon-alfa as a comparative treatment for clinical trials of new therapies against advanced renal cell carcinoma. J Clin Oncol 2002;20(1):289–96.

12. Mekhail TM, Abou-Jawde RM, Boumerhi G, et al. Validation and extension of the Memorial Sloan-Kettering prognostic factors model for survival in patients with previously untreated metastatic renal cell carcinoma. J Clin Oncol 2005;23(4):832–41.

13. Heng DY, Xie W, Regan MM, et al. Prognostic factors for overall survival in patients with metastatic renal cell carcinoma treated with vascular endothelial growth factor-targeted agents: results from a large, multicenter study. J Clin Oncol 2009;27(34):5794–9.

14. Heng DY, Xie W, Regan MM, et al. External validation and comparison with other models of the International Metastatic Renal-Cell Carcinoma Database Consortium prognostic model: a population-based study. Lancet Oncol 2013;14(2):141–8.

15. Negrier S, Escudier B, Gomez F, et al. Prognostic factors of survival and rapid progression in 782 patients with metastatic renal carcinomas treated by cytokines: a report from the Groupe Francais d'Immunotherapie. Ann Oncol 2002;13(9):1460–8.

16. Manola J, Royston P, Elson P, et al. Prognostic model for survival in patients with metastatic renal cell carcinoma: results from the International Kidney Cancer Working Group. Clin Cancer Res 2011; 17(16):5443–50.

17. Ljungberg B, Landberg G, Alamdari FI. Factors of importance for prediction of survival in patients with metastatic renal cell carcinoma, treated with or without nephrectomy. Scand J Urol Nephrol 2000;34(4):246–51.

18. Vickers MM, Al-Harbi H, Choueiri TK, et al. Prognostic factors of survival for patients with metastatic renal cell carcinoma with brain metastases treated with targeted therapy: results from the International Metastatic Renal Cell Carcinoma Database Consortium. Clin Genitourin Cancer 2013;11(3): 311–5.

19. McKay RR, Kroeger N, Xie W, et al. Impact of bone and liver metastases on patients with renal cell carcinoma treated with targeted therapy. Eur Urol 2014; 65(3):577–84.

20. Choueiri TK, Motzer RJ. Systemic therapy for metastatic renal-cell carcinoma. N Engl J Med 2017; 376(4):354–66.

21. Flanigan RC, Salmon SE, Blumenstein BA, et al. Nephrectomy followed by interferon alfa-2b compared with interferon alfa-2b alone for metastatic renal-cell cancer. N Engl J Med 2001;345(23):1655–9.

22. Motzer RJ, Bacik J, Mazumdar M. Prognostic factors for survival of patients with stage IV renal cell carcinoma: Memorial Sloan-Kettering Cancer Center experience. Clin Cancer Res 2004;10(18 Pt 2): 6302S–3S.

23. Ko JJ, Xie W, Kroeger N, et al. The International Metastatic Renal Cell Carcinoma Database Consortium model as a prognostic tool in patients with metastatic renal cell carcinoma previously treated with first-line targeted therapy: a population-based study. Lancet Oncol 2015;16(3):293–300.

24. Kroeger N, Xie W, Lee JL, et al. Metastatic non-clear cell renal cell carcinoma treated with targeted therapy agents: characterization of survival outcome and application of the International mRCC Database Consortium criteria. Cancer 2013;119(16): 2999–3006.

25. Kim T, Zargar-Shoshtari K, Dhillon J, et al. Using percentage of sarcomatoid differentiation as a prognostic factor in renal cell carcinoma. Clin Genitourin Cancer 2015;13(3):225–30.

26. Shinohara N, Abe T. Prognostic factors and risk classifications for patients with metastatic renal cell carcinoma. Int J Urol 2015;22(10):888–97.

27. Kyriakopoulos CE, Chittoria N, Choueiri TK, et al. Outcome of patients with metastatic sarcomatoid renal cell carcinoma: results from the International Metastatic Renal Cell Carcinoma Database Consortium. Clin Genitourin Cancer 2015;13(2):e79–85.

28. Strimbu K, Tavel JA. What are biomarkers? Curr Opin HIV AIDS 2010;5(6):463–6.

29. Graham J, Dudani S, Heng DYC. Prognostication in kidney cancer: recent advances and future directions. J Clin Oncol 2018. JCO2018790147.

30. Motzer RJ, Tannir NM, McDermott DF, et al. Nivolumab plus ipilimumab versus sunitinib in advanced renal-cell carcinoma. N Engl J Med 2018;36(36):1277–90.

31. Sato Y, Yoshizato T, Shiraishi Y, et al. Integrated molecular analysis of clear-cell renal cell carcinoma. Nat Genet 2013;45(8):860–7.

32. Cancer Genome Atlas Research N. Comprehensive molecular characterization of clear cell renal cell carcinoma. Nature 2013;499(7456):43–9.

33. Carlo MI, Manley B, Patil S, et al. Genomic alterations and outcomes with VEGF-targeted therapy in patients with clear cell renal cell carcinoma. Kidney Cancer 2017;1(1):49–56.

34. Voss MH, Reising A, Cheng Y, et al. Genomically annotated risk model for advanced renal-cell carcinoma: a retrospective cohort study. Lancet Oncol 2018;19(12):1688–98.

35. Hsieh JJ, Chen D, Wang PI, et al. Genomic biomarkers of a randomized trial comparing first-line everolimus and sunitinib in patients with metastatic renal cell carcinoma. Eur Urol 2017;71(3):405–14.

36. Miao D, Margolis CA, Gao W, et al. Genomic correlates of response to immune checkpoint therapies in clear cell renal cell carcinoma. Science 2018;359(6377):801–6.

37. Pan D, Kobayashi A, Jiang P, et al. A major chromatin regulator determines resistance of tumor cells to T cell-mediated killing. Science 2018;359(6377):770–5.

38. Miao D, Margolis CA, Vokes NI, et al. Genomic correlates of response to immune checkpoint blockade in microsatellite-stable solid tumors. Nat Genet 2018;50(9):1271–81.

39. Braun DA, Ishii Y, Walsh AM, et al. Clinical validation of PBRM1 alterations as a marker of immune checkpoint inhibitor response in renal cell carcinoma. JAMA Oncol 2019. https://doi.org/10.1001/jamaoncol.2019.3158.

40. Motzer RJ, Escudier B, McDermott DF, et al. Nivolumab versus everolimus in advanced renal-cell carcinoma. N Engl J Med 2015;373(19):1803–13.

41. McDermott DF, Huseni MA, Atkins MB, et al. Clinical activity and molecular correlates of response to atezolizumab alone or in combination with bevacizumab versus sunitinib in renal cell carcinoma. Nat Med 2018;24(6):749–57.

42. Beuselinck B, Verbiest A, Couchy G, et al. Tumor molecular characteristics in patients (pts) with international metastatic renal cell carcinoma database consortium (IMDC) good (G) and intermediate/poor (I/P) risk. Ann Oncol 2018;29:viii303–31.

43. Rini BI, Huseni M, Atkins MB, et al. Molecular correlates differentiate response to atezolizumab (atezo) + bevacizumab (bev) vs sunitinib (sun): results from a phase III study (IMmotion151) in untreated metastatic renal cell carcinoma (mRCC). Ann Oncol 2018;29:viii724–5.

44. Hakimi AA, Voss MH, Kuo F, et al. Transcriptomic profiling of the tumor microenvironment reveals distinct subgroups of clear cell renal cell cancer: data from a randomized phase III trial. Cancer Discov 2019;9(4):510–25.

45. Motzer RJ, Hutson TE, Cella D, et al. Pazopanib versus sunitinib in metastatic renal-cell carcinoma. N Engl J Med 2013;369(8):722–31.

46. Flaifel A, Xie W, Braun DA, et al. PD-L1 expression and clinical outcomes to cabozantinib, everolimus, and sunitinib in patients with metastatic renal cell carcinoma: analysis of the randomized clinical trials METEOR and CABOSUN. Clin Cancer Res 2019;25(20):6080–8.

47. Choueiri TK, Escudier B, Powles T, et al. Cabozantinib versus everolimus in advanced renal-cell carcinoma. N Engl J Med 2015;373(19):1814–23.

48. Choueiri TK, Halabi S, Sanford BL, et al. Cabozantinib versus sunitinib as initial targeted therapy for patients with metastatic renal cell carcinoma of poor or intermediate risk: the alliance A031203 CABOSUN trial. J Clin Oncol 2017;35(6):591–7.

49. Motzer RJ, Penkov K, Haanen J, et al. Avelumab plus axitinib versus sunitinib for advanced renal-cell carcinoma. N Engl J Med 2019;380(12):1103–15.

50. Rini BI, Powles T, Atkins MB, et al. Atezolizumab plus bevacizumab versus sunitinib in patients with previously untreated metastatic renal cell carcinoma (IMmotion151): a multicentre, open-label, phase 3, randomised controlled trial. Lancet 2019;393(10189):2404–15.

51. Rini BI, Plimack ER, Stus V, et al. Pembrolizumab plus axitinib versus sunitinib for advanced renal-cell carcinoma. N Engl J Med 2019;380(12):1116–27.

52. Raimondi A, Sepe P, Claps M, et al. Do biomarkers play a predictive role for response to novel immunotherapeutic agents in metastatic renal cell carcinoma? Expert Opin Biol Ther 2019;19(11):1107–10.

53. Rizvi NA, Hellmann MD, Snyder A, et al. Cancer immunology. Mutational landscape determines sensitivity to PD-1 blockade in non-small cell lung cancer. Science 2015;348(6230):124–8.

54. Snyder A, Makarov V, Merghoub T, et al. Genetic basis for clinical response to CTLA-4 blockade in melanoma. N Engl J Med 2014;371(23):2189–99.

55. Van Allen EM, Miao D, Schilling B, et al. Genomic correlates of response to CTLA-4 blockade in metastatic melanoma. Science 2015;350(6257):207–11.

56. de Velasco G, Miao D, Voss MH, et al. Tumor mutational load and immune parameters across metastatic renal cell carcinoma risk groups. Cancer Immunol Res 2016;4(10):820–2.

57. Yarchoan M, Hopkins A, Jaffee EM. Tumor mutational burden and response rate to PD-1 inhibition. N Engl J Med 2017;377(25):2500–1.

58. Malouf GG, Ali SM, Wang K, et al. Genomic characterization of renal cell carcinoma with sarcomatoid dedifferentiation pinpoints recurrent genomic alterations. Eur Urol 2016;70(2):348–57.

59. Samstein RM, Lee CH, Shoushtari AN, et al. Tumor mutational load predicts survival after immunotherapy across multiple cancer types. Nat Genet 2019;51(2):202–6.

60. Mauge L, Mejean A, Fournier L, et al. Sunitinib prior to planned nephrectomy in metastatic renal cell carcinoma: angiogenesis biomarkers predict clinical outcome in the prospective phase II PREINSUT trial. Clin Cancer Res 2018;24(22):5534–42.

61. Verzoni E, Carteni G, Cortesi E, et al. Real-world efficacy and safety of nivolumab in previously-treated metastatic renal cell carcinoma, and association between immune-related adverse events and survival: the Italian expanded access program. J Immunother Cancer 2019;7(1):99.

62. Sanchez A, Furberg H, Kuo F, et al. Transcriptomic signatures related to the obesity paradox in patients with clear cell renal cell carcinoma: a cohort study. Lancet Oncol 2020;21(2):283–93.

Sequencing Therapies for Metastatic Renal Cell Carcinoma

Nazli Dizman, MD[a], Zeynep E. Arslan, MD[b], Matthew Feng[a], Sumanta K. Pal, MD[a],*

KEYWORDS

- Targeted therapy • Immunotherapy • Sequencing • RCC • Kidney cancer

KEY POINTS

- In an era of several available therapeutic options, optimal treatment sequencing is crucial to providing patients with the most effective therapy and promoting quality of life.
- In clear cell renal cell carcinoma, a combination approach with an immunotherapy backbone, such as nivolumab/ipilimumab or axitinib/pembrolizumab, has established a key role in the first-line setting. Safety and activity data support the transition to single-agent targeted therapies (cabozantinib or axitinib) in the second-line setting. Nivolumab monotherapy possesses clinical and mechanistic rationale as a second-line therapeutic option for patients treated with targeted therapies in the first-line setting.
- Programmed cell death protein 1 and programmed death-ligand 1 expression levels currently are not used to guide treatment selection in clinical practice, due to lack of supporting evidence. At present, gene expression models are being generated from large prospective clinical trial data sets.

INTRODUCTION

United States–based epidemiologic studies indicate that more than 70,000 individuals are diagnosed with renal cell carcinoma (RCC) annually, and 17% of these present with metastatic disease.[1–3] RCC encompasses several histologic subtypes that bear distinct biologic and clinical features. Clear cell RCC (ccRCC) accounts for approximately 80% of all cases whereas papillary RCC represents the second major subtype and is seen in approximately 10% to 15% of cases. Rare subtypes comprise the remaining RCC population and include chromophobe RCC, collecting duct RCC, renal medullary carcinoma, and others.[4–6] In addition, sarcomatoid histology represents up to 15% of all the RCC cases and can be seen either as an isolated entity or as sarcomatoid differentiation accompanying other histologic subtypes. Tremendous efforts have been made to individualize treatment strategies in this diverse patient population with the intent of lengthening survival while maintaining the quality of life of patients with metastatic RCC (mRCC).[7,8] Accordingly, the treatment algorithm for mRCC has changed drastically within the past 2 decades.[8,9] **Fig. 1** represents the mRCC therapeutics with regulatory approval to date and their indications.

Currently available mRCC therapies can be categorized broadly as targeted therapies and immunotherapies. Mechanistically, targeted therapies blockade tumor angiogenesis via vascular endothelial growth factor (VEGF) tyrosine kinase

[a] Department of Medical Oncology and Therapeutics Research, City of Hope Comprehensive Cancer Center, 1500 East Duarte Road, Duarte, CA 91010, USA; [b] Istanbul Medipol University Medical School, Kavacık Mah. Ekinciler Cad. No: 19, Kavacık Kavşağı, 34810 Beykoz, Istanbul, Turkey
* Corresponding author.
E-mail address: spal@coh.org

Urol Clin N Am 47 (2020) 305–318
https://doi.org/10.1016/j.ucl.2020.04.008

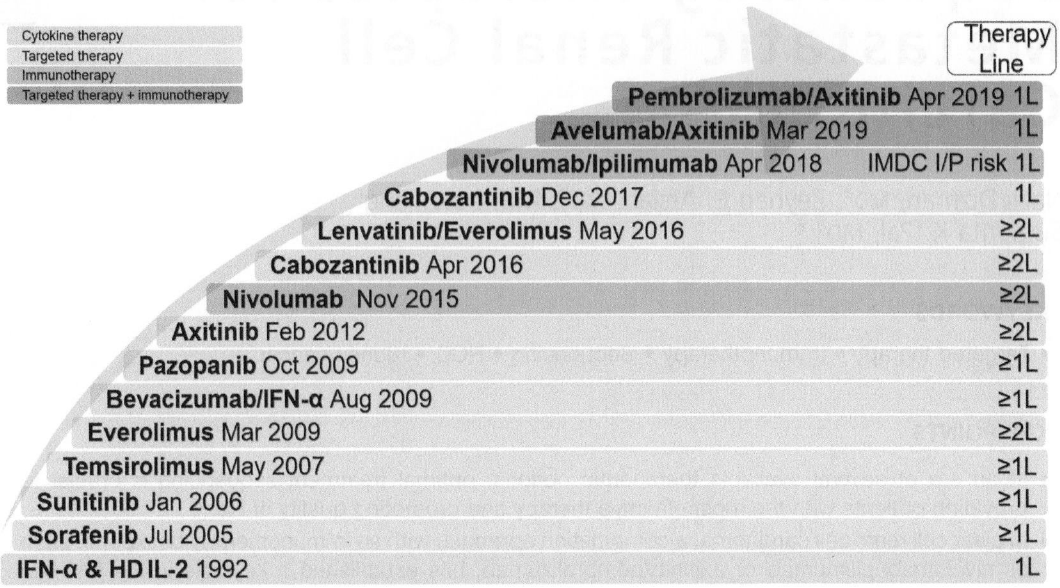

Cytokine therapy		
Targeted therapy		
Immunotherapy		
Targeted therapy + immunotherapy		

Therapy Line

Pembrolizumab/Axitinib Apr 2019		1L
Avelumab/Axitinib Mar 2019		1L
Nivolumab/Ipilimumab Apr 2018	IMDC I/P risk	1L
Cabozantinib Dec 2017		1L
Lenvatinib/Everolimus May 2016		≥2L
Cabozantinib Apr 2016		≥2L
Nivolumab Nov 2015		≥2L
Axitinib Feb 2012		≥2L
Pazopanib Oct 2009		≥1L
Bevacizumab/IFN-α Aug 2009		≥1L
Everolimus Mar 2009		≥2L
Temsirolimus May 2007		≥1L
Sunitinib Jan 2006		≥1L
Sorafenib Jul 2005		≥1L
IFN-α & HD IL-2 1992		1L

Fig. 1. Agents approved by FDA in first-line and further-line treatment of mRCC. HD, high-dose; I/P, Intermediate/Poor.

inhibitors (sunitinib, cabozantinib, axitinib, sorafenib, and pazopanib), anti-VEGF monoclonal antibodies (bevacizumab), or mammalian target of rapamycin (mTOR) inhibitors (temsirolimus and everolimus). Traditional immunotherapies, such as interferon (IFN)-α and interleukin 2, have been the mainstay of mRCC treatment in the era prior to targeted therapies. Despite moderate clinical benefit among mRCC patients, the excessive toxicities associated with traditional immunotherapies led to limitations in their utilization.[10,11] Modern immunotherapies include agents that disable tumor cells' ability to evade the immune system via inhibition of programmed cell death protein 1 (PD-1) (eg, nivolumab and pembrolizumab), programmed death-ligand 1 (PD-L1) (eg, atezolizumab and avelumab), or cytotoxic T-lymphocyte–associated protein 4 (CTLA-4) (eg, ipilimumab).[12–14] For each of these aforementioned treatment modalities, only a certain proportion of the patients have demonstrated benefit across various measurable outcomes, including progression-free survival (PFS), overall survival (OS), objective response rate (ORR), toxicity, and patient-reported outcomes. As such, all forms of treatment currently serve crucial roles in the current paradigm for the treatment of mRCC, as evidenced by the approval of 15 different therapeutic approaches, 10 agents in first-line treatment and 11 agents in further-line treatment.[7]

As the list of therapeutic options has grown, the selection of treatment among individual patients has become more challenging. Existing clinical

decision making in daily practice currently relies on assumptions based on cross-trial comparisons; however, there is a growing body of evidence regarding clinical and genomic features that potentially might guide treatment selection. For example, the CheckMate 214 study has offered insights into decision making by demonstrating benefit for International Metastatic Renal Cell Carcinoma Database Consortium (IMDC) favorable-risk patients with sunitinib and for intermediate-risk and poor-risk patients with nivolumab and ipilimumab combination as first-line treatment.[12] In addition, investigators have analyzed data from phase III trials of immunotherapy and targeted therapy combinations to develop models involving molecular characteristics and gene expression patterns of tumors to predict patients' response to therapies.[15] This article presents the current state of knowledge concerning treatment options for mRCC patients and proposes an algorithm for sequencing therapies, based on existing scientific evidence, in the hopes of prolonging survival and promoting quality of life.

CLEAR CELL RENAL CELL CARCINOMA FIRST-LINE TREATMENT OPTIONS
Targeted Therapies

The most common oncogenic event in ccRCC pathogenesis is the loss of chromosome 3p and subsequent *VHL* tumor suppressor gene alterations with either absence or malfunction of the VHL protein; hypoxia-inducible factors accumulate and prompt overexpression of growth factors, including VEGF and platelet-derived growth factor

B, culminating in tumor cell growth, proliferation, and aberrant angiogenesis. Targeted therapies that block the VEGF pathway were the first breakthrough treatment of patients with mRCC.

In 2006, Motzer and colleagues[16] reported the survival and response outcomes of first-line sunitinib versus IFN-α, with results favoring sunitinib in all major measures, including ORR, PFS, OS, and quality of life. Soon after, sunitinib was granted US Food and Drug Administration (FDA) approval, initiating a shift in the RCC treatment landscape from traditional immunotherapies (ie, high-dose interleukin and IFN-α) to the more tolerable and effective targeted therapies. Concurrently, temsirolimus, an mTOR inhibitor, showed improved PFS and OS compared with IFN-α and the combination of IFN-α and temsirolimus in patients with poor prognostic features.[17] Single-agent temsirolimus was better tolerated and provided the greatest benefit.[17] This study remains important by both demonstrating efficacy of temsirolimus in this vulnerable patient population and highlighting the value of offering a balance between efficacy and toxicity profiles during treatment planning. Pazopanib also has been utilized and evaluated widely, with initial studies among patient populations who were either treatment-naïve or pretreated with cytokine therapies.[18] Studies suggested that there was significant PFS improvement compared with placebo, results that led to a clinical trial comparing pazopanib with sunitinib in the first-line setting.[19] In this noninferiority trial, clinical outcomes were comparable between arms with PFS of 8.4 months (95% CI, 8.3–10.9) versus 9.5 months (95% CI, 8.3–11.1), respectively, and OS of 28.4 months (95% CI, 26.2–35.6) versus 29.3 months (95% CI, 25.3–32.5), respectively, for pazopanib and sunitinib.[19] The toxicity profile of pazopanib was more favorable, particularly in terms of fatigue, hand-foot syndrome, and thrombocytopenia.

The more recent next-generation targeted therapies tested in the first-line setting include axitinib, which demonstrates highly selective activity on target VEGF receptors, and cabozantinib, which inhibits multiple tyrosine kinases. Axitinib, a selective inhibitor of VEGF receptors 1, 2, and 3, failed to show a PFS improvement over sorafenib in first-line treatment.[20,21] Despite that the higher ORR with axitinib than with sorafenib might suggest activity signals, the study did not meet its primary endpoint.[21]

Evidence suggests that cabozantinib, a multikinase inhibitor of VEGF receptor, AXL, and MET, has MET and AXL receptor tyrosine kinases that are up-regulated by the accumulated hypoxia-inducible factors under pseudohypoxia conditions commonly present in RCC cells.[22,23] The combined inhibition of multikinases by cabozantinib was tested against sunitinib in the phase II CABOSUN study in first-line treatment of mRCC patients with IMDC intermediate-risk and poor-risk disease.[24,25] In a cohort of 157 mRCC patients, median PFS was 8.6 months with cabozantinib versus 5.3 months with sunitinib, per independent review committee assessment (Table 1). The difference in PFS was statistically significant, with a hazard ratio (HR) of 0.48, with 20% of patients in the cabozantinib arm achieving objective responses compared with only 9% of patients with sunitinib.[24,25] Whereas one-fifth of patients achieved an objective response in the cabozantinib arm, only 9% achieved a similar response with sunitinib. Toxicity profiles of the 2 regimens were comparable. Updated OS data after a median follow-up of 34.5 months revealed a numerical difference between the cabozantinib and sunitinib arms; however, statistical significance was not achieved.[25]

Perhaps more importantly, the results of the CABOSUN study in the patient population with bone metastases raised significant interest. Bone is the second most common metastatic site, with approximately one-third of patients developing bone metastases during the course of their mRCC progression.[14] Several studies, including a meta-analysis, have shown that bone metastasis is a poor prognostic feature for patients treated with targeted therapies.[26–28] The CABOSUN trial involved stratification and randomization based on the presence of bone metastasis, thus allowing in-depth analysis of outcomes in this vulnerable patient population. Subsequently, a significant PFS benefit was observed with cabozantinib over sunitinib in patients with bone metastasis. This elevated cabozantinib to the preferred first-line treatment option for IMDC intermediate-risk and poor-risk patients with bone involvement, per National Comprehensive Cancer Network (NCCN) guidelines.[7]

Sunitinib has remained the standard-of-care targeted therapy and main comparator arm to clinical trials in first-line mRCC treatment for more than a decade.[10,29] Development of first-line combination therapies, however, discussed later, subordinated sunitinib. In addition, the observed PFS and ORR benefits with cabozantinib over sunitinib also have encouraged the utilization of cabozantinib in first-line treatment, as opposed to sunitinib.[24] Currently, among the many available first-line targeted therapy agents, cabozantinib represents a suitable targeted therapy option, especially among immunotherapy-ineligible patients, such as those with active autoimmune disease or systemic steroid use (Fig. 2).

Table 1
Efficacy and safety outcomes in first-line clinical trials in metastatic renal cell carcinoma

	CABOSUN[24,25]	IMmotion151 (Intention-to-Treat Population)[41,42]	IMmotion 151 (Programmed Death-Ligand 1+)[41,42]	CheckMate 214 (Intention-to-Treat Population)[12]	CheckMate 214 (IMDC Favorable)[12]	CheckMate 214 (IMDC Intermediate/Poor)[12]	KEYNOTE-426[13]	JAVELIN Renal 101 (Intention-to-Treat Population)[14]	JAVELIN Renal 101 (Programmed Death-Ligand 1+)[14]
Arms	Cabozantinib vs sunitinib	Atezolizumab + bevacizumab vs sunitinib		Nivolumab + ipilimumab vs sunitinib			Pembrolizumab + axitinib vs sunitinib	Avelumab + axitinib vs sunitinib	
Accrual (N)	157	915	362	1096	249	847	861	886	560
Phase	II	III	III	III	III	III	III	III	III
Stratification factors	IMDC risk group Bone metastasis	MSKCC risk group Liver metastasis PD-L1 expression (<1% vs ≥1%)		IMDC risk group Geographic region			IMDC risk group Geographic region	ECOG performance status Geographic region	
PFS (mo)	8.6 vs 5.3	11.2 vs 8.4	11.2 vs 7.7	9.7 vs 9.7	NR vs NR	8.2 vs 8.3	15.1 vs 11.1	13.8 vs 8.4	13.8 vs 7.2
HR (95% CI)	0.48 (0.31–0.74)	0.83 (0.70–0.97)	0.74 (0.57–0.96)	0.85 (0.73–0.98)	1.23 (0.90–1.69)	0.77 (0.65–0.90)	0.69 (0.57–0.84)	0.69 (0.56–0.84)	0.61 (0.47–0.79)
P value	P = .0008	P = .0219	P = .0217	P = .027	P = .19	P = .0014	P<.001	P<.001	P<.001
OS (mo)	26.6 vs 21.2	33.6 vs 34.9	34.0 vs 32.7	NR vs 37.9	NR vs NR	NR vs 26.6	89.9% vs 78.3% at 12 mo	NE	NE
HR (95% CI)	0.80 (0.53–1.21)	0.93 (0.76–1.14)	0.84 (0.62–1.15)	0.71 (0.59–0.86)	1.22 (0.73–2.04)	0.66 (0.54–.080)	0.53 (0.38–0.74)		
P value		P = .4751	P = .2857	P = .0003	P = .44	P<.0001	P<.0001		
ORR (%)	20 vs 9	37 vs 33	43 vs 35	41 vs 34	39 vs 50	42 vs 29	59.3 vs 35.7	51.4 vs 25.7	55.2 vs 5.5
Complete response (%)	0 vs 0	5 vs 2	9 vs 4	11 vs 2	8 vs 4	11 vs 1	5.8 vs 1.9	3.4 vs 1.8	4.4 vs 2.1

Partial response (%)	20 vs 9	31 vs 31	34 vs 30	31 vs 32	31 vs 46	31 vs 28	53.5 vs 33.8	48 vs 23.9	50.7 vs 3.4
Stable disease (%)	54 vs 38	39 vs 39	32 vs 35	30 vs 41	44 vs 39	26 vs 41	24.5 vs 39.4	29.6 vs 45.5	26.7 vs 3.1
Progressive disease (%)	18 vs 29	18 vs 19	19 vs 21	22 vs 16	12 vs 5	25 vs 19	10.9 vs 17	11.5 vs 18.7	11.1 vs 1.7
NE (%)	8 vs 23	7 vs 9	7 vs 10	7 vs 10	5 vs 6	7 vs 10	1.9 vs 1.4	5.7 vs 7.9	4.4 vs 7.2
Adverse events									
All grade (%)	92 vs 89	91 vs 96		81 vs 83			98.4 vs 99.5	99.5 vs 99.3	
Grade 3–4 (%)	68 vs 65	40 vs 54		47 vs 64			62.9 vs 58.1	71.2 vs 71.5	
Treatment discontinuation (%)	21 vs 22	5 (both), 2 (atezolizumab), 5 (bevacizumab) vs 8		22 vs 12[a]			10.7 (both), 30.5 (either) vs 13.9	7.6 (both) vs 13.4	

Abbreviations: ECOG, Eastern Cooperative Oncology Group; NE, not evaluable; NR, not reached.

[a] 29% received ≥40-mg prednisone.

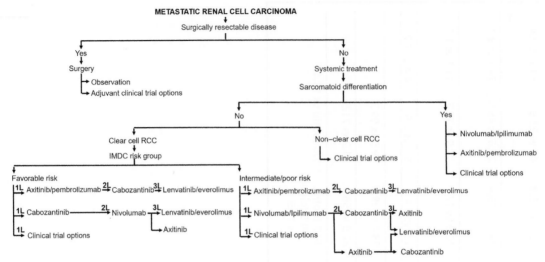

Fig. 2. Authors' proposed management algorithm for patients with mRCC.

Immunotherapies

In addition to possessing angiogenic characteristics, RCC bears high immunogenicity.[15,30] Traditional immunotherapies, cytokines, had been the mainstay of mRCC treatment in the era prior to targeted therapies. By the early 2000s, identification of immune checkpoint molecules, such as CTLA-4 and PD-1 on the surface of T cells and PD-L1 on dendritic cells and tumor cells, restored scientific interest in immuno-oncology agents.[31] In the realm of RCC therapeutics, the PD-1 inhibitor, nivolumab, was the first immunotherapy to establish activity, with better OS outcomes and tolerability over everolimus in patients who failed on treatment with a targeted therapy.[32]

The immuno-oncology approach later was adopted in the first-line setting as part of a more aggressive strategy, including a combination nivolumab and ipilimumab in the phase III CheckMate 214 clinical trial.[12] The results of this study brought essential insights on the efficacy of immunotherapeutics in mRCC.[12] In total, 1096 treatment-naïve mRCC patients were enrolled and received either a combination of nivolumab and ipilimumab or single-agent sunitinib (see **Table 1**).[12] Randomization was stratified based on IMDC risk categories (favorable risk vs intermediate–high risk) and geographic region.[12] The treatment regimen in the combination arm employed administration of nivolumab, 3 mg/kg, and ipilimumab, 1 mg/kg, every 3 weeks for 4 courses, and then maintenance nivolumab, 3 mg/kg, every 2 weeks, whereas a traditional treatment schedule was used in the sunitinib arm, with 50 mg/d orally, with 4 weeks on 2 weeks off.[12]

The initial results of 25 months follow-up revealed notable activity of the combination over sunitinib in a patient population with IMDC intermediate-risk or high-risk disease. OS was not reached in the combination arm versus 26 months in the sunitinib arm. Moreover, HR for death was 0.63, reflecting a 37% reduction of risk of death with the combination agent, and the 18-month OS rates were 75% and 60% in the combination arm and the sunitinib arm, respectively.[12] PFS accordingly was longer in the combination arm, but the difference was not statistically significant (11.6 months vs 8.4 months; HR 0.82; 99.1% CI, 0.64–1.05). Response rates favored the combination treatment, with ORRs of 42% and 27%, respectively, with 9% of the patients experiencing a complete response in the immunotherapy arm versus 1% in the sunitinib arm.[12] Direction of benefit, however, was the inverse in the favorable-risk patient population; the 18-month OS rate was 88% with combination therapy and 93% with sunitinib and demonstrated an HR of 1.45 (99.8% CI, 0.51–4.12).[12] Median PFS was 15.3 months in the combination arm versus 25.1 months in the sunitinib arm (HR 2.18; 99.1% CI, 1.29–3.68), and ORR was 29% with the combination versus 52% with sunitinib.[12] Importantly, the combination of nivolumab and ipilimumab provided a complete response in 11% of the patients in the favorable-risk population, whereas only 6% achieved a similar response with sunitinib.

Updated outcomes of the CheckMate 214 trial, after a minimum follow-up of 42 months, have confirmed the sustained OS and ORR benefits associated with this combination therapy in intermediate-risk and poor-risk populations.[33] In addition, over this extended follow-up period, the difference in PFS between the combination arm and the sunitinib arm increased and reached statistical significance (12.0 months vs 8.3 months, respectively; HR 0.76 [0.63–0.91]). In the overall population, the 42-month OS rate was 56% in the combination arm versus 47% with sunitinib, recording a P value of 0.0002. Similar to the results of the initial analyses, a median OS was not reached and the difference between arms was not significant in the favorable-risk patient group. The combination of nivolumab and ipilimumab demonstrated higher complete response rates over sunitinib in the overall cohort, intermediate–poor-risk disease cohort, and favorable-risk cohort, with rates of 11% versus 2%, respectively; 10% versus 1%, respectively; and 13% versus 6%, respectively. Notably, 86% of complete responses were ongoing at the time of data cutoff, and 28 of the 59 complete responders did not require a subsequent treatment after discontinuation of nivolumab and ipilimumab after a median duration of 34.6 months.

Concerning safety outcomes, both all-grade and grade 3–4 adverse events were seen more frequently in the sunitinib arm. Despite this, treatment discontinuation due to adverse events was more common with immunotherapy (22%) than sunitinib (12%), patient-reported outcomes reported by Cella and colleagues[34] suggested better tolerability of the immunotherapy combination over sunitinib.[12]

The substantial survival benefit and the longevity of the responses observed with nivolumab and ipilimumab combination led to approval of the combination agents for metastatic ccRCC patients with IMDC intermediate-risk and poor-risk patients. The NCCN and Society for Immunotherapy of Cancer (SITC) guidelines now recommend nivolumab and ipilimumab combination as preferred treatment in metastatic ccRCC patients with IMDC intermediate-risk or poor-risk disease.[7,35]

Importantly, the contrasting benefit patterns in different IMDC risk classes with 2 mechanistically distinct approaches brought about a new perspective to the field. IMDC risk classification originally was developed as a prognostic tool among a large cohort of mRCC patients receiving targeted therapy.[36] Benefit from immunotherapy in this patient population, which was previously identified as bearing poor prognosis, extended this domain of investigation to identifying molecular correlates of response to immunotherapies. The CheckMate 214 study included exploratory analyses of clinical outcomes based on PD-L1 expression; however, among the intermediate-risk and high-risk cohorts, OS benefit with the immunotherapy combination over sunitinib was independent of PD-L1 expression levels.[12] When a positive PD-L1 expression level was defined by greater than or equal to 1%, ORR favored immunotherapy in both PD-L1–positive and PD-L1–negative patients.[12] Therefore, the predictive capability of PD-L1 expression was considered inconclusive and possibly not clinically significant with the nivolumab and ipilimumab combination.

Pembrolizumab also was studied in the first-line treatment of mRCC in the phase II Keynote-427 study.[37] An analysis of the 107 enrolled patients demonstrated efficacy with ORR of 33.6% and the treatment had favorably safety.[13] Single-agent pembrolizumab has not been investigated further, however, given the profound efficacy of combination therapy involving pembrolizumab in first-line treatment of mRCC, data that are discussed later. Single-agent immunotherapy currently is not considered appropriate first-line therapy.

Instead, combination nivolumab and ipilimumab is a standard-of-care option for immunotherapy-eligible patients with IMDC intermediate-risk and poor-risk disease (see **Fig. 2**).

Combination Therapies

Following the success of targeted therapies and immunotherapies in mRCC treatment, further efforts were directed to evaluating combination therapies that could inhibit angiogenesis and foster immune surveillance simultaneously.[13,14] Investigators sought to attain immediate decreases in tumor burden with PFS benefit, combined with durable responses and OS benefit, with a favorable toxicity profile. In addition, basic science research showed that targeted therapies bear immunomodulatory effects within the tumor microenvironment by prompting regulatory T cells, myeloid-derived suppressor cells, and cytokines to suppress ongoing immune escape.[38–40] Thus, a combination of the two active compounds could possess a potential synergistic activity beyond their additive effects.

The randomized phase III IMmotion151 trial was the first to report outcomes of the combination approach in first-line treatment of mRCC patients with clear cell or sarcomatoid histology (see **Table 1**).[41] The study enrolled 915 patients randomized to sunitinib or a combination of bevacizumab and atezolizumab. Stratification factors included PD-L1 expression (<1% vs ≥1%) on tumor-infiltrating lymphocytes, presence of liver metastasis, and Memorial Sloan Kettering Cancer Center (MSKCC) prognostic group.[41] Median PFS in the

PD-L1–positive population and in the intention-to-treat population both favored the bevacizumab/atezolizumab combination over sunitinib (11.2 months vs 7.7 months, respectively, HR 0.74; and 11.2 months vs 8.4 months, respectively, HR 0.83). OS was comparable, however, across both arms in both PD-L1–positive and the intention-to-treat analyses.[41] In this study, important results emerged among those with sarcomatoid histology[42]; 61% of patients with sarcomatoid histology were PD-L1–positive and there was substantial improvement observed in ORR and PFS when those patients were treated with bevacizumab/atezolizumab.[42] In the PD-L1–positive sarcomatoid RCC patients, PFS results favored bevacizumab/atezolizumab, with an HR of 0.46. More importantly, the superior efficacy of bevacizumab/atezolizumab in terms of ORR and PFS was independent from PD-L1 status among sarcomatoid RCC patients.[42] Despite that, the IMmotion151 trial met its first coprimary endpoint, the PFS benefit in a PD-L1–positive patient population, the second co-primary endpoint of OS benefit in the overall population was not met, and thus the combination has not received regulatory approval.

Two other breakthrough studies in the realm of mRCC treatment were reported in 2019; the KEYNOTE-426 and JAVELIN Renal 101 trials (see **Table 1**). KEYNOTE-426 compared the combination of pembrolizumab and axitinib with sunitinib, whereas JAVELIN Renal 101 compared the combination of avelumab and axitinib with sunitinib.[13,14] Both combinations obtained immediate FDA approval within months. In the KEYNOTE-426 study, pembrolizumab and axitinib met primary endpoints of OS and PFS along with the key secondary endpoint of ORR.[13] At the 12-month cutoff of OS analysis, 89.9% versus 78.3% of the patients were alive in the combination and sunitinib arms, respectively.[13] The statistical difference favored pembrolizumab/axitinib with an HR of 0.53. Median PFS was 15.1 months in the pembrolizumab/axitinib arm versus 11.1 months in the sunitinib arm. In the combination arm, 59.3% of the patients achieved an objective response, with 5.8% having complete response; in contrast, ORR was 35.7% and only 1.9% of the patients achieved complete response in the sunitinib arm.[13] The randomization of the study was stratified based on IMDC risk status of patients, and the results showed that OS and PFS benefits with the combination were independent of IMDC risk status or PD-L1 expression status.

In the JAVELIN Renal 101 study, the combination of avelumab and axitinib demonstrated improved PFS over sunitinib in both the PD-L1 positive ($\geq$1% on immune cells) and overall population (13.8 months vs 7.2 months, respectively [HR 0.61; 95% CI, 0.47–0.79], and 13.8 months vs 8.4 months, respectively [HR 0.69; 95% CI, 0.56–0.84].[14] In the overall population, ORR was 51.4% with the combination treatment versus 25.7% with sunitinib, with complete response rates of 3.4% and 1.8%, respectively. At the time of the first publication, OS data of the study were not mature and only a small number of patients were deceased in each group.[14]

When evaluating the results of the 2 FDA-approved combination therapies involving a targeted therapy and immunotherapy, toxicity profile becomes an important area of consideration. The proportions of the patients who developed any grade adverse event appeared comparable in KEYNOTE-426 and JAVELIN Renal 101, 98.4% and 95.4%, respectively, with 10.7% and 7.6%, respectively, of patients requiring discontinuation of the combination due to side effects.[13,14] Rates of fatigue, hypertension, and rash were similar in both combination therapies. The combination of pembrolizumab/axitinib was associated with a higher rate of hypothyroidism (35.4% vs 24.9%) and gastrointestinal toxicities, such as diarrhea (62.2% vs 54.3%) and nausea (34.1% vs 27.7%) compared with avelumab/axitinib. Overall, the toxicity profiles of the pembrolizumab/axitinib and avelumab/axitinib were similar.

Whereas both combinations obtained almost immediate FDA approval, most current guidelines of NCCN and SITC both recommend pembrolizumab/axitinib as the preferred immunotherapy-targeted therapy combination in the first-line setting, regardless of IMDC risk category, due primarily to the lack of OS data in the JAVELIN 101 clinical trial.[7,35] The authors' preferences are in line with these guideline recommendations (see **Fig. 2**).

FURTHER-LINE TREATMENT

Decisions regarding second-line treatment strategies are based broadly on the type of first-line therapeutic a patient has received. According to a large 2014 study, VEGF–tyrosine kinase inhibitors were the agents utilized most commonly by US-based medical oncologists for patients with RCC.[43] Although the results of this report might now be outdated with addition of the novel immunotherapeutics and combination therapies, there remains a considerable number of patients who received or have been receiving first-line targeted therapies. Second-line options for this patient population include single-agent nivolumab or 1 of the other targeted therapies, including mTOR inhibitors or VEGF-directed therapies. Details of clinically relevant second-line and further-line studies are presented in **Table 2**.

For patients who had been treated with first-line targeted therapies, nivolumab represents a sensible option based on the results of the CheckMate 025 study, wherein nivolumab was compared with everolimus in targeted therapy–exposed mRCC patients.[32,44] In this study, approximately two-thirds of patients had received sunitinib, whereas the remaining received pazopanib or axitinib prior to the study therapy. Median OS was reached at 25 months (95% CI, 21.8-NE) with nivolumab

compared with 19.6 months (95% CI, 17.6–23.1) with everolimus, with HR of death of 0.73 (98.5% CI, 0.57–0.93). OS benefit with nivolumab remained significant within different subgroups of patients with regard to IMDC risk stratification, age, metastatic sites, and type of prior targeted therapeutic.[32,44] Importantly, forest plots showed more prominent benefit with nivolumab in patients with IMDC poor-risk disease. Whereas PFS was similar between the 2 cohorts, a notable 25% of the patients had objective response in the nivolumab arm versus 5% in the everolimus arm.[32,44] In light of the results of CheckMate 025, the most

Table 2
Outcomes in clinical trials examining second-line and further-line therapies in metastatic renal cell carcinoma

	Axitinib vs Sorafenib[20]	Lenvatinib + Everolimus vs Lenvatinib vs Everolimus[54]	Nivolumab vs Everolimus[32]	Cabozantinib vs Everolimus[51]
Accrual (N)	723	153	821	658
Phase	III	II	III	III
PFS (mo) HR (95% CI) P value	8.3 vs 5.7 0.66 (0.55–0.78) P<.0001	14.6 vs 7.4 vs 5.5 0.40 (0.24–0.68) P = .005[a] 0.66 (0.39–1.10) P = .12[b] 0.61 (0.38–0.98) P = .048[c]	4.6 vs 4.4 0.88 (0.75–1.03) P = .11	7.4 vs 3.8 0.58 (0.45–0.75) P<.001
OS (mo) HR (95% CI) P value	20.1 vs 19.2 0.97 (0.80–1.17) P = .374	25.5 vs 19.1 vs 15.4 0.51 (0.30–0.88) P = .024[a] 0.75 (0.43–1.30) P = .32[b] 0.68 (0.41–1.14) P = .12[c]	25 vs 19.6 0.73 (0.57–0.93) P = .002	21.4 vs 16.5 0.66 (0.53–0.83) P = .00026
ORR (%) P value	19 vs 11 P = .0007	43 vs 27 vs 6[a] P<.0001[a] P = .10[b] P = .0067[c]	25 vs 5 P<.001	17 vs 3 P<.0001
Complete response (%)	0 vs <1	2 vs 0 vs 0	1 vs <1	0 vs 0
Partial response (%)	19 vs 11	41 vs 27 vs 6	24 vs 5	17 vs 3
Stable disease (%)	58 vs 59	41 vs 52 vs 62	34 vs 55	65 vs 62
Progressive disease (%)	17 vs 18	4 vs 6 vs 21	35 vs 28	12 vs 27
Not evaluable (%)	7 vs 11	12 vs 15 vs 8	6 vs 12	5 vs 8
Adverse events				
All grade (%)	NA vs NA	99 vs 94 vs 96	79 vs 88	100 vs 100
Grade 3–4 (%)	NA vs NA	71 vs 79 vs 50	19 vs 37	71 vs 60
Treatment discontinuation (%)	4 vs 8	24 vs 25 vs 12	8 vs 13	12 vs 11

Abbreviation: NA, not available.
[a] Lenvatinib and everolimus versus everolimus.
[b] Lenvatinib and everolimus versus lenvatinib.
[c] Lenvatinib versus everolimus.

current guidelines of NCCN and SITC recommend nivolumab as a preferred subsequent-line treatment, for those who progressed on first-line targeted therapies.[7,35]

Due to the increasing number of patients receiving first-line combination therapy involving 2 immunotherapeutics or an immunotherapeutic and a VEGF-directed therapy, second-line treatment selection after progression on first-line combinations is an emerging and increasingly critical issue. At present, there have been no published studies prospectively evaluating the efficacy of individual subsequent therapies, and thus the current state of knowledge is based on the retrospective reports in the literature.[45–49] Overall, studies examining this question have revealed efficacy and safety of VEGF-directed therapies after both immunotherapy doublet and immunotherapy and VEGF-directed therapy combinations.[45–49] For example, Dudani and colleagues[49] examined the IMDC cohort and reported outcomes with second-line targeted therapies after immunotherapy combinations. A total of 188 patients were included in the analysis, of which 113 patients were treated with first-line immunotherapy and targeted therapy combination and the remainder with nivolumab and ipilimumab. Response rates, OS rates, and times to treatment failure were similar between the 2 cohorts. Dudani and colleagues[49] carefully analyzed the clinical outcomes associated with subsequent therapies after combination therapy and revealed several hypothesis-generating results. Response to subsequent-line targeted therapies was higher in patients who received first-line nivolumab and ipilimumab than in those who received an immunotherapy and VEGF-directed therapy combination (45% versus 15%, respectively; $P = .040$), whereas times to treatment failure were 5.4 months and 3.7 months, respectively, although this latter difference was not statistically significant.[49]

As demonstrated in **Fig. 1**, in addition to nivolumab, several targeted therapy options exist in the treatment of mRCC patients after failure of first-line therapy. The NCCN kidney cancer guidelines recommend cabozantinib, axitinib, or lenvatinib/everolimus combination as preferred and category 1 targeted therapy in second-line and further-line settings.[7] Unfortunately, due to the unparalleled development and utilization of novel first-line combinations, no prospective evidence exists concerning the comparative efficacy of individual targeted therapies after novel first-line combinations. Recommendations on treatment sequencing in this state are based largely on studies testing the aforementioned agents in targeted therapy–treated patients. **Table 2** represents the results of the clinical trials testing mentioned therapies.

Cabozantinib represents a widely used and studied option in second-line setting of mRCC. Preclinical studies have revealed that previous sunitinib treatment enhances invasive ability of RCC cells and accelerates tumor growth. Blockade of MET and AXL via cabozantinib was shown to decrease tumor size and overcome the sunitinib-induced aggressive characteristics in xenograft models.[50] In parallel with this strong biologic rationale, cabozantinib has demonstrated improvement in 3 endpoints, PFS, OS, and ORR, compared with everolimus, in a population of patients treated previously with targeted therapies.[51] Subgroup analyses in this trial showed sustained efficacy for both OS and PFS outcomes regardless of IMDC groups, MET status of tumors, number of the prior therapies, and metastatic sites.[51] Importantly, for patients with bone metastases, cabozantinib represented an appropriate option with subgroup analyses favoring cabozantinib in patients with bone metastases. Regarding the post-immunotherapy efficacy of cabozantinib, a retrospective analysis showed disease control rates of 82% in patients exposed to prior-line immunotherapy and 75% in patients with previous treatment of immunotherapy and targeted therapy combination.[52] Thus, either after a combination therapy involving either 2 immunotherapies or an immunotherapy and targeted therapy, cabozantinib is a better option due to its mechanistic rationale and clinical evidence (see **Fig. 2**).

The next generation of clinical trials in the realm of mRCC will need to prioritize addressing issues in sequencing therapies under standardized conditions. The phase III PDIGREE trial (NCT03793166) has taken an important step to elucidate the sequencing strategies with immunotherapies and cabozantinib. In this ongoing clinical trial, patients with IMDC intermediate-risk or high-risk metastatic ccRCC are enrolled and initiated on nivolumab and ipilimumab combination. Following a preplanned management strategy based on treatment response, patients with progressive disease are switched to cabozantinib, whereas patients with complete response continue with single-agent nivolumab maintenance therapy. Patients who do not progress but do not achieve a complete response are randomized into either nivolumab maintenance therapy alone or in combination with cabozantinib. The PDIGREE trial aims to maximize treatment benefit by upscaling treatment strategies for those without an objective response and sparing responders from side effects of unnecessarily aggressive treatment combinations and offers the potential to address various questions regarding treatment sequencing.

Axitinib has been introduced to the arena with a promising safety profile due to its highly selective inhibition of VEGF receptors. The profound antitumor activity of axitinib was demonstrated by significant PFS and ORR benefit over sorafenib in the second-line setting.[21] The number of adverse events seen with axitinib appeared similar to agents of the same therapeutic class, and side effects generally were more manageable. In addition, in this trial, the investigators included and periodically obtained the objective measures of symptom burden (Functional Assessment of Cancer Therapy–Kidney Symptom Index [FKSI] questionnaire and FKSI–Disease-related Symptoms subscale) as endpoints, with results revealing that symptom deterioration was significantly delayed in the axitinib arm compared with the sorafenib arm.[21] More recently, Ornstein and colleagues[53] published the phase II clinical data of axitinib in a novel dosing schedule that allowed dose adjustments based on side effects in a patient population previously treated with immune checkpoint inhibitors. This novel dosing scheme demonstrated the manageability of side effects associated with axitinib, with individualized dose adjustments or interruptions, without compromising efficacy. In detail, the novel schedule provided ORR of 20%, with an additional 50% of the patients possessing stable disease and a median PFS of 8.8 months. Importantly, none of the patients in this study required permanent treatment discontinuation due to adverse events.[53] Accordingly, for all patients after first-line nivolumab and ipilimumab treatment, or for fragile patients in further lines of therapy, axitinib would be a logical next step given the evident efficacy and tolerability (see **Fig. 2**).

The combination of lenvatinib and everolimus gained approval based on the results of a phase II clinical trial comparing the combination with single-agent everolimus, an mTOR inhibitor, and single-agent lenvatinib.[54] The combination exhibited better OS and PFS compared with single-agent everolimus but failed to show a statistically significant difference over single-agent lenvatinib with regard to OS and PFS (see **Table 2**).[54] Importantly, the combination of lenvatinib and everolimus provided ORR of 43%, with an additional 41% of patients experiencing disease stabilization. In light of the findings of this phase II study, the FDA approved the lenvatinib/everolimus combination in the treatment of targeted therapy–treated mRCC patients. Efforts currently are under way to explore the efficacy of this combination with a lower dose of lenvatinib in a phase II clinical trial (NCT03173560) in postimmunotherapy or post-targeted therapy setting and to compare the combination with sunitinib or a combination of pembrolizumab and lenvatinib (NCT02811861) in first-line setting.

Given that the evidence about the efficacy of this combination currently relies on phase II clinical trial data and the lack of benefit supporting superiority of the combination over lenvatinib in terms of PFS and OS, the authors consider the lenvatinib/everolimus combination as a further treatment option after failure on second-line cabozantinib or axitinib.

For patients who progressed on more than 2 therapies, the reliability of comparative evidence gradually decreases. In current clinical practice, utilization of next-generation sequencing emerges as a preferred approach to identify targetable genomic alterations.[55] Next-generation sequencing can be implemented in clinical practice through various commercial platforms that sequence tumor tissue specimens obtained by surgical interventions or biopsies or on circulating tumor DNA (ctDNA) extracted from a blood sample (ie, liquid biopsy).[55,56] Despite the fact that such alterations are not as highly predictive as in other solid cancer types, such as *EGFR* in non–small cell lung cancer or *BRAF* in melanoma, a growing body of evidence in mRCC points to certain associations with prognosis and prediction of benefit from therapies. For example, *PBRM1* mutations were found to be good prognostic indicators overall and to possess sensitivity to immunotherapies.[57,58] *BAP1* mutations have been associated with worse prognostic features, whereas alterations in genes contributing to mTORC1 signaling (ie, *MTOR*, *TSC1*, *TSC2*, and *PIK3CA*) were associated with enhanced benefit from mTOR inhibitors.[59–61] Evolution of tumor genomic characteristics with exposure to therapeutics also deserves attention. Sequential ctDNA assessment of 220 mRCC patients during their disease course yielded changes in rates of genomic alterations by time, suggesting a rationale for repeat screening for formation of new genomic alterations.[62] Ongoing investigations analyzing genomic findings of patients participating in large clinical trials are promising to provide better predictive markers to help personalize therapeutic approaches in both first line and subsequent lines of mRCC treatment.

SUMMARY

Within the past 2 decades, the mRCC treatment landscape has been rapidly revolutionized with the development of novel therapeutics, such as targeted therapies, immunotherapies, and combination approaches. As a result, mRCC patients now have the potential to achieve longer survival durations without experiencing detrimental treatment side effects. Sequencing available therapies in a way that would enable a balance of survival benefit and toxicity profile is crucial. For ccRCC patients or for those with sarcomatoid histology, a combination therapy with an immunotherapy backbone, such as nivolumab and ipilimumab or pembrolizumab and axitinib, has established a role in front-line treatment, with evidence of improved PFS, OS, and ORR compared with single-agent targeted therapy. For those with contraindications for immunotherapies, cabozantinib provides a beneficial option with observed PFS and ORR benefit over sunitinib. The selection of subsequent lines of treatment largely relies on the mechanistic category of prior line of therapy. Second-line nivolumab is the recommended approach for immunotherapy-naïve patients. Following failure of nivolumab and ipilimumab, further options include a sequence of cabozantinib and axitinib, which is guided by available retrospective activity and tolerability data. Cabozantinib represents an appropriate option after progression on pembrolizumab and axitinib.

DISCLOSURE

S.K. Pal reports consulting for Genentech, Aveo, Eisai, Roche, Pfizer, Novartis, Exelixis, Ipsen, BMS, and Astellas. N. Dizman, Z.E. Arslan, and M. Feng declare no conflict of interests.

REFERENCES

1. Leibovich BC, Blute ML, Cheville JC, et al. Prediction of progression after radical nephrectomy for patients with clear cell renal cell carcinoma: a stratification tool for prospective clinical trials. Cancer 2003;97: 1663–71.
2. Siegel RL, Miller KD, Jemal A. Cancer statistics, 2020. CA Cancer J Clin 2020;70:7–30.
3. Capitanio U, Bensalah K, Bex A, et al. Epidemiology of Renal Cell Carcinoma. Eur Urol 2019;75(74–84).
4. Moch H, Cubilla AL, Humphrey PA, et al. The 2016 WHO classification of tumours of the urinary system and male genital organs-part a: renal, penile, and testicular tumours. Eur Urol 2016;70:93–105.
5. Muglia VF, Prando A. Renal cell carcinoma: histological classification and correlation with imaging findings. Radiol Bras 2015;48:166–74.
6. Ricketts CJ, De Cubas AA, Fan H, et al. The Cancer Genome Atlas Comprehensive Molecular Characterization of Renal Cell Carcinoma. Cell Rep 2018;23: 313–26.e5.
7. Jonasch E. NCCN guidelines updates: management of metastatic kidney cancer. J Natl Compr Canc Netw 2019;17:587–9.
8. Escudier B. Combination therapy as first-line treatment in metastatic renal-cell carcinoma. N Engl J Med 2019;380:1176–8.
9. Brugarolas J. Renal-cell carcinoma–molecular pathways and therapies. N Engl J Med 2007;356:185–7.
10. Cohen HT, McGovern FJ. Renal-Cell Carcinoma. New Engl J Med 2005;353:2477–90.
11. Koneru R, Hotte SJ. Role of cytokine therapy for renal cell carcinoma in the era of targeted agents. Curr Oncol 2009;16:S40–4.
12. Motzer RJ, Tannir NM, McDermott DF, et al. Nivolumab plus ipilimumab versus sunitinib in advanced renal-cell carcinoma. N Engl J Med 2018;378: 1277–90.
13. Rini BI, Plimack ER, Stus V, et al. Pembrolizumab plus axitinib versus sunitinib for advanced renal-cell carcinoma. N Engl J Med 2019;380:1116–27.
14. Motzer RJ, Penkov K, Haanen J, et al. Avelumab plus axitinib versus sunitinib for advanced renal-cell carcinoma. N Engl J Med 2019;380: 1103–15.
15. Choueiri TK, Albiges L, Haanen JBAG, et al. Biomarker analyses from JAVELIN Renal 101: Avelumab + axitinib (A+Ax) versus sunitinib (S) in advanced renal cell carcinoma (aRCC). J Clin Oncol 2019;37:101.
16. Motzer RJ, Hutson TE, Tomczak P, et al. Sunitinib versus interferon alfa in metastatic renal-cell carcinoma. N Engl J Med 2007;356:115–24.
17. Hudes G, Carducci M, Tomczak P, et al. Temsirolimus, interferon alfa, or both for advanced renal-cell carcinoma. N Engl J Med 2007;356:2271–81.
18. Sternberg CN, Davis ID, Mardiak J, et al. Pazopanib in locally advanced or metastatic renal cell carcinoma: results of a randomized phase III trial. J Clin Oncol 2010;28:1061–8.
19. Motzer RJ, Hutson TE, Cella D, et al. Pazopanib versus sunitinib in metastatic renal-cell carcinoma. N Engl J Med 2013;369:722–31.
20. Rini BI, Escudier B, Tomczak P, et al. Comparative effectiveness of axitinib versus sorafenib in advanced renal cell carcinoma (AXIS): a randomised phase 3 trial. Lancet 2011;378:1931–9.
21. Hutson TE, Lesovoy V, Al-Shukri S, et al. Axitinib versus sorafenib as first-line therapy in patients with metastatic renal-cell carcinoma: a randomised open-label phase 3 trial. Lancet Oncol 2013;14: 1287–94.
22. Nakaigawa N, Yao M, Baba M, et al. Inactivation of von Hippel-Lindau gene induces constitutive phosphorylation of MET protein in clear cell renal carcinoma. Cancer Res 2006;66:3699–705.
23. Rankin EB, Fuh KC, Castellini L, et al. Direct regulation of GAS6/AXL signaling by HIF promotes renal

metastasis through SRC and MET. Proc Natl Acad Sci U S A 2014;111:13373–8.

24. Choueiri TK, Halabi S, Sanford BL, et al. Cabozantinib versus sunitinib as initial targeted therapy for patients with metastatic renal cell carcinoma of poor or intermediate risk: the alliance A031203 CABOSUN Trial. J Clin Oncol 2017;35:591–7.

25. Choueiri TK, Hessel C, Halabi S, et al. Cabozantinib versus sunitinib as initial therapy for metastatic renal cell carcinoma of intermediate or poor risk (Alliance A031203 CABOSUN randomised trial): Progression-free survival by independent review and overall survival update. Eur J Cancer 2018;94:115–25.

26. McKay RR, Kroeger N, Xie W, et al. Impact of bone and liver metastases on patients with renal cell carcinoma treated with targeted therapy. Eur Urol 2014; 65:577–84.

27. Motzer RJ, Escudier B, Bukowski R, et al. Prognostic factors for survival in 1059 patients treated with sunitinib for metastatic renal cell carcinoma. Br J Cancer 2013;108:2470–7.

28. Beuselinck B, Oudard S, Rixe O, et al. Negative impact of bone metastasis on outcome in clear-cell renal cell carcinoma treated with sunitinib. Ann Oncol 2011;22:794–800.

29. Choueiri TK, Motzer RJ. Systemic Therapy for Metastatic Renal-Cell Carcinoma. N Engl J Med 2017; 376:354–66.

30. McDermott DF, Huseni MA, Atkins MB, et al. Clinical activity and molecular correlates of response to atezolizumab alone or in combination with bevacizumab versus sunitinib in renal cell carcinoma. Nat Med 2018;24:749–57.

31. Egen JG, Allison JP. Cytotoxic T Lymphocyte Antigen-4 Accumulation in the Immunological Synapse Is Regulated by TCR Signal Strength. Immunity 2002;16:23–35.

32. Motzer RJ, Escudier B, McDermott DF, et al. Nivolumab versus everolimus in advanced renal-cell carcinoma. N Engl J Med 2015;373:1803–13.

33. Tannir NM, McDermott DF, Escudier B, et al. Overall survival and independent review of response in CheckMate 214 with 42-month follow-up: First-line nivolumab + ipilimumab (N+I) versus sunitinib (S) in patients (pts) with advanced renal cell carcinoma (aRCC). J Clin Oncol 2020;38:609.

34. Cella D, Grünwald V, Escudier B, et al. Patient-reported outcomes of patients with advanced renal cell carcinoma treated with nivolumab plus ipilimumab versus sunitinib (CheckMate 214): a randomised, phase 3 trial. Lancet Oncol 2019;20: 297–310.

35. Rini BI, Battle D, Figlin RA, et al. The Society for Immunotherapy of Cancer consensus statement on immunotherapy for the treatment of advanced renal cell carcinoma (RCC). J Immunother Cancer 2019;7: 354.

36. Heng DYC, Xie W, Regan MM, et al. Prognostic factors for overall survival in patients with metastatic renal cell carcinoma treated with vascular endothelial growth factor-targeted agents: results from a large, multicenter study. J Clin Oncol 2009;27: 5794–9.

37. McDermott DF, Lee J-L, Szczylik C, et al. Pembrolizumab monotherapy as first-line therapy in advanced clear cell renal cell carcinoma (accRCC): Results from cohort A of KEYNOTE-427. J Clin Oncol 2018;36:4500.

38. Ozao-Choy J, Ma G, Kao J, et al. The novel role of tyrosine kinase inhibitor in the reversal of immune suppression and modulation of tumor microenvironment for immune-based cancer therapies. Cancer Res 2009;69:2514–22.

39. Xin H, Zhang C, Herrmann A, et al. Sunitinib inhibition of Stat3 induces renal cell carcinoma tumor cell apoptosis and reduces immunosuppressive cells. Cancer Res 2009;69:2506–13.

40. Finke JH, Rini B, Ireland J, et al. Sunitinib reverses type-1 immune suppression and decreases T-regulatory cells in renal cell carcinoma patients. Clin Cancer Res 2008;14:6674–82.

41. Rini BI, Powles T, Atkins MB, et al. Atezolizumab plus bevacizumab versus sunitinib in patients with previously untreated metastatic renal cell carcinoma (IMmotion151): a multicentre, open-label, phase 3, randomised controlled trial. Lancet 2019;393: 2404–15.

42. Rini BI, Motzer RJ, Powles T, et al. Atezolizumab (atezo) + bevacizumab (bev) versus sunitinib (sun) in pts with untreated metastatic renal cell carcinoma (mRCC) and sarcomatoid (sarc) histology: IMmotion151 subgroup analysis. J Clin Oncol 2019;37: 4512.

43. Jonasch E, Signorovitch JE, Lin PL, et al. Treatment patterns in metastatic renal cell carcinoma: a retrospective review of medical records from US community oncology practices. Curr Med Res Opin 2014; 30:2041–50.

44. Escudier B, Sharma P, McDermott DF, et al. CheckMate 025 randomized phase 3 study: outcomes by key baseline factors and prior therapy for nivolumab versus everolimus in advanced renal cell carcinoma. Eur Urol 2017;72:962–71.

45. Dizman N, Bergerot PG, Bergerot CD, et al. Targeted therapies following first-line immune checkpoint inhibitor combination in metastatic renal cell carcinoma: a single center experience. Kidney Cancer 2019;3:171–6.

46. Barata PC, Gomez de Liano A, Mendiratta P, et al. Clinical outcome of patients (Pts) with metastatic renal cell carcinoma (mRCC) progressing on front-line immune-oncology based combination (IO-COMBO) regimens. J Clin Oncol 2018;36: 613.

47. Shah AY, Kotecha RR, Lemke EA, et al. Outcomes of patients with metastatic clear-cell renal cell carcinoma treated with second-line VEGFR-TKI after first-line immune checkpoint inhibitors. Eur J Cancer 2019;114:67–75.

48. Auvray M, Auclin E, Barthelemy P, et al. Second-line targeted therapies after nivolumab-ipilimumab failure in metastatic renal cell carcinoma. Eur J Cancer 2019;108:33–40.

49. Dudani S, Graham J, Wells JC, et al. First-line immuno-oncology combination therapies in metastatic renal-cell carcinoma: results from the international metastatic renal-cell carcinoma database consortium. Eur Urol 2019;76:861–7.

50. Zhou L, Liu X-D, Sun M, et al. Targeting MET and AXL overcomes resistance to sunitinib therapy in renal cell carcinoma. Oncogene 2016;35:2687–97.

51. Choueiri TK, Escudier B, Powles T, et al. Cabozantinib versus Everolimus in Advanced Renal-Cell Carcinoma. N Engl J Med 2015;373:1814–23.

52. McGregor BA, Lalani A-K, Xie W, et al. Activity of cabozantinib (cabo) after PD-1/PD-L1 immune checkpoint blockade (ICB) in metastatic clear cell renal cell carcinoma (mccRCC). Ann Oncol 2018;29:viii311.

53. Ornstein MC, Pal SK, Wood LS, et al. Individualised axitinib regimen for patients with metastatic renal cell carcinoma after treatment with checkpoint inhibitors: a multicentre, single-arm, phase 2 study. Lancet Oncol 2019;20:1386–94.

54. Motzer RJ, Hutson TE, Glen H, et al. Lenvatinib, everolimus, and the combination in patients with metastatic renal cell carcinoma: a randomised, phase 2, open-label, multicentre trial. Lancet Oncol 2015;16:1473–82.

55. Hsieh JJ, Le V, Cao D, et al. Genomic classifications of renal cell carcinoma: a critical step towards the future application of personalized kidney cancer care with pan-omics precision. J Pathol 2018;244:525–37.

56. Bergerot PG, Hahn AW, Bergerot CD, et al. The Role of Circulating Tumor DNA in Renal Cell Carcinoma. Curr Treat Options Oncol 2018;19:10.

57. Miao D, Margolis CA, Gao W, et al. Genomic correlates of response to immune checkpoint therapies in clear cell renal cell carcinoma. Science 2018;359:801–6.

58. Voss MH, Reising A, Cheng Y, et al. Genomically annotated risk model for advanced renal-cell carcinoma: a retrospective cohort study. Lancet Oncol 2018;19:1688–98.

59. Kapur P, Peña-Llopis S, Christie A, et al. Effects on survival of BAP1 and PBRM1 mutations in sporadic clear-cell renal-cell carcinoma: a retrospective analysis with independent validation. Lancet Oncol 2013;14:159–67.

60. Joseph RW, Kapur P, Serie DJ, et al. Loss of BAP1 protein expression is an independent marker of poor prognosis in patients with low-risk clear cell renal cell carcinoma. Cancer 2014;120:1059–67.

61. Kwiatkowski DJ, Choueiri TK, Fay AP, et al. Mutations in TSC1, TSC2, and MTOR are associated with response to rapalogs in patients with metastatic Renal Cell Carcinoma. Clin Cancer Res 2016;22:2445–52.

62. Pal SK, Sonpavde G, Agarwal N, et al. Evolution of circulating tumor DNA profile from first-line to subsequent therapy in metastatic renal cell carcinoma. Eur Urol 2017;72:557–64.

Management of Metastatic Renal Cell Carcinoma with Variant Histologies

Ronan Flippot, MD[a,c], Vijay Damarla, MD[b], Bradley A. McGregor, MD[a],*

KEYWORDS

- Non–clear cell renal cell carcinoma • Immune checkpoint inhibitors • Tyrosine kinase inhibitors

KEY POINTS

- Variant histology renal cell carcinoma (vRCC) encompasses various entities with different molecular features.
- Systemic therapies in patients with metastatic vRCC are generally less active than in patients with conventional clear-cell renal cell carcinoma.
- Cytoreductive nephrectomy in the metastatic setting should be considered on a case-by-case basis for vRCC considering the lack of prospective data.
- Therapies targeting angiogenesis have shown substantial response rates, but comparative trials are lacking for these rare tumors.
- Immune checkpoint inhibitors are being evaluated as monotherapy or combination with early evidence of durable benefit. Ongoing trials are underway and may further improve outcomes of patients with vRCC.

INTRODUCTION

Renal cell carcinoma (RCC) affects more than 400,000 patients worldwide, and half of these patients will ultimately harbor metastatic disease.[1] Most RCC are of the clear cell (ccRCC) subtype, characterized by alterations of *VHL* and subsequent activation of the hypoxia-inducible factor pathway, as well as chromatin remodeling genes *BAP1*, *PBRM1*, and *SETD2*. Conversely, up to 25% of RCCs belong to the heterogeneous group of non–clear cell RCC, or variant histology renal cell carcinoma (vRCC), which encompasses diseases with different biology and distinct natural history. The most frequent subtypes of vRCC include papillary, chromophobe, collecting duct, renal medullary carcinomas, Xp11 translocation carcinomas, and succinate dehydrogenase deficient renal carcinomas, some of which may occur in the context of familial predisposition syndromes (**Table 1**).[2]

vRCCs are generally associated with aggressive metastatic behavior, decreased survival, and poor response to treatment with targeted molecular therapies compared with conventional clear cell tumors.[3] Advances in the molecular characterization of vRCC and the surge of immunotherapy-based regimens have paved the way for new therapeutic developments that may durably improve outcomes of patients with vRCC. Herein the authors discuss the biological landscape of vRCC and review current and future therapeutic options for patients with metastatic vRCC.

[a] Dana-Farber Cancer Institute, Lank Center for Genitourinary Oncology, 450 Brookline Avenue, Boston, MA 02215, USA; [b] Decatur Memorial Hospital, 2300 North Edward Street, Decatur, IL 62526, USA; [c] Department of Cancer Medicine, Gustave Roussy, 114 rue Edouard Vaillant, Villejuif 94800, France
* Corresponding author.
E-mail address: bradley_mcgregor@dfci.harvard.edu

Urol Clin N Am 47 (2020) 319–327
https://doi.org/10.1016/j.ucl.2020.04.003
0094-0143/20/© 2020 Elsevier Inc. All rights reserved.

Table 1
Main biological alterations in variant histology renal cell carcinoma

RCC Type	Chromosomal Alterations	Main Molecular Alterations	Main Familial Predispositions
Papillary type I	Gain of chromosome 7, 17, deletion of 1p36	*MET*	Hereditary pRCC (*MET*)
Papillary type II	Loss of chromosome 9p21, 3p	*CDKN2A*, *SETD2*, BAP1, PBRM1, activation of NRF2-ARE, TFE3 fusions	HLRCC (*FH*)
Chromophobe	Loss of chromosome 1, 2, 6, 10, 13, 17, and 21	*TP53, PTEN, mTOR, TERT*	Birt-Hogg-Dubé syndrome (*FLCN*)
Collecting duct	DNA losses at 8p, 16p, 1p and 9p; gains at 13q	Mitochondrial genome alterations	
Renal medullary carcinoma		*SMARCB1*	Sickle cell trait
Xp11 translocation carcinoma	*TFE3* or *TFEB* rearrangements	*BIRC7* expression	

MAIN BIOLOGICAL FEATURES OF VARIANT HISTOLOGY RENAL CELL CARCINOMA

Papillary renal cell carcinoma (pRCC) is the most frequent type of vRCC and comprises 15% to 20% of all RCCs. These tumors had been further divided histologically into pRCC types 1 and 2, but the latter group actually encompasses tumors with heterogeneous biology.[2] Clinical behavior of pRCC ranges from indolent localized tumors to aggressive metastatic subtypes more frequently encountered in type 2 histologies.[4] Recurrent alterations in type 1 pRCC include gain of chromosome 7 and mutations of *MET*(7q31), present in 81% of tumors.[5] Molecular characterization of type 2 pRCC identified a diverse set of alterations to include high activation of the NRF2 antioxidant response pathway, *CDKN2A* alterations (25%) conferring adverse outcomes, CpG island methylator phenotype associated with early and aggressive onset, silencing of *CDKN2A* and frequent *FH* mutations, as well as mutations in chromatin modifying genes *SETD2*, *BAP1*, and *PBRM1*.[4]

Chromophobe renal cell carcinoma (chRCC) is the second most frequent vRCC, accounting for ~5% of all RCCs, and is notably characterized by mitochondrial alterations, multiple losses of heterozygosity involving chromosomes 1, 2, 6, 10, 13, 17, and 21, as well as *TP53* (33% to 58%) and *PTEN* mutations (9% to 24%).[6,7]

Rare variants of vRCC encompass the most aggressive tumors, which often result from single somatic driver mutations and occur earlier in life. Those include translocation RCC, characterized by rearrangements of the MiTF family transcription factors *TFE3* and *TFEB*, accounting for aggressive diseases arising in young patients; collecting duct carcinoma, notable for metabolic alterations as well as *CDKN2A* and Hippo member *NF2* alterations; and renal medullary carcinoma, in which loss of the chromatin remodeling gene *SMARCB1* has been identified as the main driver alteration.[8]

On top of molecular alterations that could foster the development of targeted molecular therapies, new data have emerged about the immunology of vRCC. These tumors generally feature infiltration by mononuclear cells and frequent programmed death-ligand 1 (PD-L1) expression on both tumor cells and tumor infiltrating immune cells.[9,10] As such, many types of vRCC appear to be immunogenic tumors and potentially amenable to therapeutic strategies based on immune checkpoint inhibitors.

THE ROLE OF NEPHRECTOMY IN METASTATIC VARIANT HISTOLOGY RENAL CELL CARCINOMA

Cytoreductive nephrectomy (CN) has long been standard of care in the management of advanced RCC based on data from SWOG 8949 and EORTC 30947, which compared interferon-α with or without nephrectomy in metastatic ccRCC.[11,12] However, the benefit in overall survival (OS) demonstrated in these trials[12] was not confirmed in the era of targeted molecular therapy. The CAR-MENA trial evaluated sunitinib versus immediate CN followed by sunitinib in patients with intermediate- or poor-risk ccRCC. This study enrolled 450 patients and showed a median OS of 18.4 months with sunitinib alone compared with 13.9 months in the CN arm, demonstrating noninferiority of sunitinib alone.[13]

However, in the setting of vRCC, where therapy is less effective, the role of CN continues to be controversial. Notably, a retrospective study from the International Metastatic RCC Database Consortium (IMDC) showed that CN was associated with improved survival in advanced RCC patients (20.6 vs 9.5 months), including 196 patients with vRCC (15.3 vs 8.0 months).[14] Additional data in 353 pRCC revealed a similar OS benefit (16.3 vs 8.6 months),[15] whereas a study based on the Surveillance, Epidemiology, and End Results database between 2001 and 2014 in 851 advanced vRCC showed a reduction in 2-year cancer-specific mortality from 77% to 52.6% with a CN.[16] Considering the lack of prospective data in vRCC, the role of CN remains unsettled and should be discussed on a case-by-case basis. Data from ccRCC trials suggest that upfront CN may especially benefit patients with low extrarenal tumor burden and good performance status, as well as those with significant symptoms from the primary tumor.[17]

SYSTEMIC THERAPY FOR VARIANT HISTOLOGY RENAL CELL CARCINOMA
Targeted Molecular Therapies

Development of systemic therapies in vRCC has largely followed the management of ccRCC. Notably, several trials evaluating VEGFR-TKIs demonstrated some activity in vRCC (**Table 2**), but their activity pales in comparison to that in ccRCC, because survival remains commonly less than 18 months.[18] Two randomized phase 2 trials, ASPEN and ESPN, were conducted in a selected vRCC population to evaluate the VGFR-TKI sunitinib versus the mTOR inhibitor everolimus in the metastatic setting.[19,20] The ASPEN trial demonstrated a significant increase in median progression-free survival (PFS) in patients treated with sunitinib compared with everolimus (8.3 vs 5.6 months), but the effect seemed to differ between prognostic risk groups and histology. Indeed, median PFS was numerically superior with everolimus compared with sunitinib in patients with poor-risk tumors, as well as in patients with chRCC. There was no difference in OS between arms. ESPN included patients with vRCC or ccRCC with greater than 20% sarcomatoid features and did not show any difference in median PFS between sunitinib (6.1 months) and everolimus (4.1 months). Median OS was 16.2 months

and 14.9 months in the sunitinib and everolimus groups, respectively.[20] Two additional randomized trials evaluated mTOR inhibitors in an unselected RCC population, including vRCC. The RECORD-3 trial evaluated the sequence sunitinib-everolimus versus everolimus-sunitinib and included 14% of patients with vRCC, in whom OS was similar between both arms, at 16.8 versus 16.2 months, respectively.[21] Finally, GLOBAL-ARCC evaluated temsirolimus versus interferon-α or both and included 20% of patients with vRCC, showing a median OS of 11.6 months with temsirolimus compared with 4.3 months with interferon-α in this population.[22,23]

These data established sunitinib as the preferred option for patients with advanced vRCC in clinical practice, although efficacy remains limited as suggested by other single-arm phase 2 trials showing objective response rates (ORR) less than 15% regardless of histology.[24,25] Prospective studies have since been reported for pazopanib and axitinib, hinting at more promising efficacy data. In 29 patients with advanced vRCC treated with pazopanib, of whom 66% harbored a papillary histology, 28% of patients responded and median PFS was 16.5 months.[26] A phase 2 trial of axitinib in 40 patients with advanced vRCC who had progressed on temsirolimus demonstrated a ORR of 37.5% with a median PFS of 7.4 months.[27] In another phase 2 trial including 44 patients with pRCC only, axitinib provided an ORR of 28.6% and a median PFS of 6.6 months.[28] Although the data are retrospective, cabozantinib is active in vRCC and is intriguing particularly in papillary subtypes given its MET inhibition. In a multicenter retrospective review of 112 patients, cabozantinib exhibited a response rate of 27% across vRCC subtypes with a median time to treatment failure of 6.7 months and a 12-month OS of 51%.[29]

Combinations of targeted molecular therapies have also been evaluated, showing interesting results in subsets of patients. The combination of everolimus with bevacizumab showed interesting activity and was well tolerated in 35 patients with advanced vRCC, including mostly papillary and unclassified tumors.[30] The overall response rate (ORR) was 29%, with a median PFS of 11 months and a median OS of 18.5 months in these aggressive tumor subtypes. The combination of erlotinib and bevacizumab has also been evaluated in sporadic pRCC as well as pRCC associated with hereditary leiomyomatosis and renal cell cancer (HLRCC), based on the alleged activity of erlotinib on tumor cell metabolism.[31] In this trial, ORR was 44% for the whole cohort (N = 41).[32,33] Importantly, ORR was up to 60% in the cohort of

Table 2
Results of selected prospective clinical trials in variant histology renal cell carcinoma

Clinical Trial	Treatment	Line of Treatment	Number of Patients Enrolled	Histology	ORR, %	PFS, mo	OS, mo
SUPAP[24]	Sunitinib	First line	61	pRCC	13 (type I) and 11 (type II)	6.6 (type I) and 5.5 (type II)	17.8 (type I) and 12.4 (type II)
RAPTOR[49]	Everolimus	First line	88	Metastatic pRCC	1	7.9 (type I) and 5.1 (type II)	28 (type I) and 24.2 (type II)
ESPN[20]	Sunitinib vs everolimus	First line	68	vRCC and ccRCC with >20% sarcomatoid features	9 vs 3	6.1 vs 4.1	16.2 vs 14.9
ASPEN[19]	Sunitinib vs everolimus	First line	108	vRCC	18 vs 9	8.3 vs 5.6	31.5 vs 13.2
RECORD-3[21]	Sunitinib-everolimus vs everolimus-sunitinib	First line	66/238 (vRCC/total)	vRCC and ccRCC	—	7.2 vs 5.1	16.8 vs 16.2
GLOBAL ARCC[22]	Temsirolimus vs interferon-α	First line	124/626 (vRCC/total)	vRCC and ccRCC	5 vs 8	7 vs 1.8	11.6 vs 4.3
Choueiri et al,[34] 2017	Savolitinib	Any line	109	pRCC	7	6.2 (MET driven) and 1.4 (MET independent)	—
KEYNOTE 427 (cohort B)[43]	Pembrolizumab	First line	165	vRCC	25	4.1	Not reached
McGregor et al,[44] 2019	Atezolizumab and bevacizumab	Any line	60	vRCC and ccRCC with >20% sarcomatoid features	33	8.3	Not reached

Abbreviation: ORR, objective response rate.

patients with HLRCC (N = 20), with a median PFS up to 24.2 months, establishing a compelling therapeutic option in these patients.

Recent efforts have aimed at MET, a recurrent driver in pRCC.[5] A biomarker-based, single-arm, phase 2 trial of the MET inhibitor savolitinib was conducted in 109 patients with metastatic pRCC, of whom 40% had driver alterations of *MET*.[34] MET-driven pRCC achieved significantly increased ORR (18% vs 0%) and median PFS (6.2 vs 1.4 months) compared with MET-independent pRCC, confirming antitumor activity of savolitinib in MET-driven tumors. Foretinib, a multikinase inhibitor of MET, AXL, and VEGFR, demonstrated antitumor activity in advanced pRCC, with median PFS of 9.3 months and ORR of 13.5% in a phase 2 single-arm trial.[35] Crizotinib, which inhibits MET, ALK, and ROS-1, provided 2 partial responses and 1 stable disease in 4 patients with MET-driven pRCC.[36] Tivantinib, developed as a selective MET inhibitor, was studied either alone or in combination with erlotinib but failed to show antitumor activity in either arm, leading to early discontinuation.[37] Although early results from the savolitinib and crizotinib trials could have foreshadowed a promising future for MET inhibitors in pRCC, phase 3 trials with these agents have been stopped prematurely. Indeed, the phase 3 trial SAVOIR comparing sunitinib to savolitinib in pRCC was discontinued because of slow enrollment, whereas the PAPMET trial comparing sunitinib to savolitinib, crizotinib, or cabozantinib prematurely closed the crizotinib and savolitinib arms. As such, targeting driver alterations in vRCC remains a challenge for future therapeutic developments.

Immune Checkpoint Inhibitors

Considering the current limitations of targeted molecular therapies in vRCC, the need for novel therapeutic strategies is essential in poor-risk patients. The alleged immunogenicity of these tumors[9] suggests that immune checkpoint inhibitors could take a leading role in the future management of vRCC.

Although the anti–programmed cell death-1 (PD-1) antibody nivolumab has been Food and Drug Administration approved since 2015 in ccRCC after demonstrating survival advantage over sunitinib in the second-line setting,[38] data on PD-1/PD-L1 inhibition in vRCC have been scant (see **Table 2**). A retrospective analysis of 41 patients with vRCC from 6 US cancer centers treated with nivolumab revealed encouraging activity with partial responses in 20%, although more than 50% had progressive disease as best response.[39]

Accumulating further evidence, another retrospective study including 40 patients with vRCC or ccRCC with greater than 20% rhabdoid features treated with nivolumab showed a response rate of 22%, including 9% complete responses, with a median PFS of 4.9 months and a median OS of 21.7 months.[40] These results were particularly encouraging because these patients were heavily pretreated with up to 8 lines of previous anticancer therapies. Additional datasets confirmed response rates of up to 20%, predominantly in pRCC and translocation RCC, as well as in patients who did not receive prior lines of therapy.[41] One retrospective study confirmed some evidence of activity for PD-1/PD-L1 inhibitors in translocation RCC, with a 17% objective response rate in 24 patients regardless of lines of therapy.[42]

The cohort B of the KEYNOTE-427 trial, a single-arm, open-label, phase 2 study of pembrolizumab monotherapy in treatment-naïve advanced vRCC, was the first study to prospectively assess the efficacy of PD-1 inhibition in vRCC.[43] A total of 165 patients with previously untreated vRCC were included and received pembrolizumab every 3 weeks for 2 years or until progression or withdrawal. Main subsets of vRCC were papillary (71%), chromophobe (13%), and unclassified (16%). At a median follow-up of 11.1 months, 56% of patients discontinued pembrolizumab because of either progression or withdrawal. The response rate was 24.8%, including 8 complete responses and 33 partial responses, with different outcomes according to histologic subtype: 34.6% of patients with unclassified RCC had objective response, compared with 25.4% for pRCC and 13% for chRCC. However, response rates were similar between patients with favorable IMDC risk (28.3%) and patients with intermediate or poor IMDC risk (23.3%). Expression of PD-L1 on tumor and immune cells as measured through Freeman antibody appeared to impact efficacy, because the response rate was 33.3% in patients with a combined positive score ≥ 1 compared with 10.3% in patients with a combined positive score less than 1.[43]

Combinations of immune checkpoint inhibitors with other approved therapies aim to improve these promising results. The anti–PD-L1 antibody atezolizumab has been evaluated in combination with the anti-VEGF antibody bevacizumab in a phase 2 trial including 60 patients with either vRCC or ccRCC with greater than 20% sarcomatoid features,[44] who may have received previous systemic therapy (35%). Response rate was 26% in those patients with vRCC (N = 42). Median PFS was 8.3 months in the entire cohort, with a median time to response of 2.7 months (range

Table 3
Selected ongoing clinical trials including variant histology renal cell carcinoma

Clinical Trial	Study Design	Treatment	Histology	Primary Endpoint	Secondary Endpoint
NCT02761057 (PAPMET)	Phase 2, randomized	Cabozantinib, crizotinib, savolitinib, sunitinib	Metastatic papillary renal carcinoma	PFS	ORR, OS
NCT03091192 (SAVOIR)	Phase 3, randomized	Savolitinib, sunitinib	MET-driven metastatic pRCC	PFS	OS, ORR
NCT01130519	Phase 2, single arm	Bevacizumab and erlotinib	HLRCC, sporadic papillary cancer	ORR	PFS, OS, DOR
NCT02495103	Phase 1/2, nonrandomized	Vandetanib and metformin	HLRCC, SDH-associated RCC, sporadic pRCC	Safety, ORR	—
NCT03541902 (CABOSUN 2)	Phase 2, randomized	Cabozantinib, sunitinib	vRCC	PFS	ORR, OS
NCT03354884 (BONSAI)	Phase 2, single arm	Cabozantinib	Collecting duct RCC	ORR	PFS, OS
NCT03635892	Phase 2, single arm	Nivolumab and cabozantinib	vRCC	ORR	—
NCT03177239 (UNISoN)	Phase 2 single arm, sequential	Nivolumab followed by nivolumab and ipilimumab	vRCC	ORR	DOR, PFS
NCT03203473 (OMNIVORE)	Phase 2, nonrandomized	Nivolumab, ipilimumab	ccRCC and vRCC	Persistent PR or CR after discontinuation PD or SD that converts to PR or CR at 1 y with addition of ipilimumab	PFS, OS

Abbreviation: DOR, duration of response ; ORR, objective reponse rate.

1.2–11.1) and a median duration of response of 8.9 months (range 1.4–29). Median OS was not reached after a median follow-up of 13 months. In an exploratory analysis of 36 patients with archival tissue available for testing, PD-L1 expression on tumor cells appeared to be associated with response: 60% in patients with PD-L1 expression ≥1%, compared with 19% in PD-L1–negative patients. In addition, there was a phase 2 trial combining the anti–PD-L1 antibody durvalumab with savolitinib in patients with pRCC stratified according to PD-L1 and MET status.[45] Although responses were shown in 27% of patients, neither PD-L1 expression (cutoff >25% on immune cells) nor MET status was predictive of response or survival. More combinations of immune checkpoint inhibitors with or without TKI are currently under investigation in vRCC and have the potential to enter clinical practice in the near future (**Table 3**).

PERSPECTIVES

An improved understanding of vRCC has been made possible thanks to molecular characterization and identification of various oncogenic processes associated with distinct entities. However, translating these understandings into new therapeutic options is a work in progress. CN can continue to be considered in the management of vRCC given the lower efficacy of current systemic therapies. Targeted therapies and immune checkpoint inhibitors, alone or in combination, appear to be steadily improving outcomes of patients despite a lack of randomized trials, which are technically more challenging in this context of rare tumors. Reports of complete responses to immune checkpoint inhibitors have been particularly encouraging[46] and support the use of immunotherapy alone or in combination with VEGF inhibitors in the upfront management of RCC. Further collaborative efforts are needed to consent patients to larger-scale trials and study biomarkers of response to therapy. Ongoing trials exploring immunotherapy combinations and targeted approaches will be critical to advance the care of vRCC (see **Table 3**).

Biomarker-based trials, such as those evaluating MET inhibitors, have been plagued by poor accrual and early termination, although results are awaited from PAPMET. Additional work is needed to investigate potential predictors of response to immune checkpoint inhibitors. Although PD-L1 expression in vRCC has been reported to be associated with response to both immune checkpoint inhibitor monotherapy and combination with VEGF inhibitors, heterogeneity in its assessments as well as clinical benefit in

PD-L1–negative patients raise questions about its applicability in clinical practice.[43,44] Gene expression signatures developed in ccRCC[47,48] and levels of lymphocyte infiltration[10] could potentially be useful for defining the immunogenic context of vRCC subtypes and identify tumors that could best benefit from immunotherapy-based approaches.

Ultimately, the promise of individualized treatment of patients with vRCC is yet to be fulfilled. However, it has become a burgeoning research field with active trials of several new therapeutic options that could yet provide durable benefit to these underserved patients.

ACKNOWLEDGMENTS

The authors acknowledge Kevin Pels for his assistance in preparing the article.

REFERENCES

1. Bray F, Ferlay J, Soerjomataram I, et al. Global cancer statistics 2018: GLOBOCAN estimates of incidence and mortality worldwide for 36 cancers in 185 countries. CA Cancer J Clin 2018;68(6): 394–424.
2. Moch H, Cubilla AL, Humphrey PA, et al. The 2016 WHO classification of tumours of the urinary system and male genital organs–part A: renal, penile, and testicular tumours. Eur Urol 2016;70(1):93–105.
3. Kroeger N, Xie W, Lee J-L, et al. Metastatic non-clear cell renal cell carcinoma treated with targeted therapy agents: characterization of survival outcome and application of the International mRCC Database Consortium Criteria. Cancer 2013;119(16): 2999–3006.
4. Cancer Genome Atlas Research Network, Linehan WM, Spellman PT, Ricketts CJ, et al. Comprehensive molecular characterization of papillary renal-cell carcinoma. N Engl J Med 2016;374(2):135–45.
5. Albiges L, Guegan J, Le Formal A, et al. MET is a potential target across all papillary renal cell carcinomas: result from a large molecular study of pRCC with CGH array and matching gene expression array. Clin Cancer Res 2014;20(13):3411–21.
6. Davis CF, Ricketts CJ, Wang M, et al. The somatic genomic landscape of chromophobe renal cell carcinoma. Cancer Cell 2014;26(3):319–30.
7. Casuscelli J, Weinhold N, Gundem G, et al. Genomic landscape and evolution of metastatic chromophobe renal cell carcinoma. JCI Insight 2017;2(12) [pii:92688].
8. Albiges L, Flippot R, Rioux-Leclercq N, et al. Non-clear cell renal cell carcinomas: from shadow to light. J Clin Oncol 2018. https://doi.org/10.1200/JCO.2018.79.2531. JCO2018792531.

9. Choueiri TK, Fay AP, Gray KP, et al. PD-L1 expression in nonclear-cell renal cell carcinoma. Ann Oncol 2014;25(11):2178–84.

10. Flippot R, McGregor BA, Flaifel A, et al. Atezolizumab plus bevacizumab in non-clear cell renal cell carcinoma (NccRCC) and clear cell renal cell carcinoma with sarcomatoid differentiation (ccRCCsd): updated results of activity and predictive biomarkers from a phase II study. J Clin Oncol 2019;37(15_suppl):4583.

11. Flanigan RC, Salmon SE, Blumenstein BA, et al. Nephrectomy followed by interferon alfa-2b compared with interferon alfa-2b alone for metastatic renal-cell cancer. N Engl J Med 2001;345(23):1655–9.

12. Flanigan RC, Mickisch G, Sylvester R, et al. Cytoreductive nephrectomy in patients with metastatic renal cancer: a combined analysis. J Urol 2004; 171(3):1071–6.

13. Méjean A, Ravaud A, Thezenas S, et al. Sunitinib alone or after nephrectomy in metastatic renal-cell carcinoma. N Engl J Med 2018;379(5):417–27.

14. Heng DYC, Wells JC, Rini BI, et al. Cytoreductive nephrectomy in patients with synchronous metastases from renal cell carcinoma: results from the International Metastatic Renal Cell Carcinoma Database Consortium. Eur Urol 2014;66(4):704–10.

15. Graham J, Wells JC, Donskov F, et al. Cytoreductive nephrectomy in metastatic papillary renal cell carcinoma: results from the International Metastatic Renal Cell Carcinoma Database Consortium. Eur Urol Oncol 2019;2(6):643–8.

16. Marchioni M, Bandini M, Preisser F, et al. Survival after cytoreductive nephrectomy in metastatic non-clear cell renal cell carcinoma patients: a population-based study. Eur Urol Focus 2019;5(3): 488–96.

17. Mejean A, Thezenas S, Chevreau C, et al. Cytoreductive nephrectomy (CN) in metastatic renal cancer (mRCC): update on Carmena trial with focus on intermediate IMDC-risk population. J Clin Oncol 2019;37(15_suppl):4508.

18. Vera-Badillo FE, Templeton AJ, Duran I, et al. Systemic therapy for non-clear cell renal cell carcinomas: a systematic review and meta-analysis. Eur Urol 2015;67(4):740–9.

19. Armstrong AJ, Halabi S, Eisen T, et al. Everolimus versus sunitinib for patients with metastatic non-clear cell renal cell carcinoma (ASPEN): a multicentre, open-label, randomised phase 2 trial. Lancet Oncol 2016;17(3): 378–88.

20. Tannir NM, Jonasch E, Albiges L, et al. Everolimus versus sunitinib prospective evaluation in metastatic non-clear cell renal cell carcinoma (ESPN): a randomized multicenter phase 2 trial. Eur Urol 2016; 69(5):866–74.

21. Knox JJ, Barrios CH, Kim TM, et al. Final overall survival analysis for the phase II RECORD-3 study of first-line everolimus followed by sunitinib versus first-line sunitinib followed by everolimus in metastatic RCC. Ann Oncol 2017;28(6):1339–45.

22. Hudes G, Carducci M, Tomczak P, et al. Temsirolimus, interferon alfa, or both for advanced renal-cell carcinoma. N Engl J Med 2007;356(22): 2271–81.

23. Dutcher JP, de Souza P, McDermott D, et al. Effect of temsirolimus versus interferon-alpha on outcome of patients with advanced renal cell carcinoma of different tumor histologies. Med Oncol 2009;26(2): 202–9.

24. Ravaud A, Oudard S, De Fromont M, et al. First-line treatment with sunitinib for type 1 and type 2 locally advanced or metastatic papillary renal cell carcinoma: a phase II study (SUPAP) by the French Genitourinary Group (GETUG)†. Ann Oncol 2015;26(6): 1123–8.

25. Tannir NM, Plimack E, Ng C, et al. A phase 2 trial of sunitinib in patients with advanced non-clear cell renal cell carcinoma. Eur Urol 2012;62(6):1013–9.

26. Jung KS, Lee SJ, Park SH, et al. Pazopanib for the treatment of non-clear cell renal cell carcinoma: a single-arm, open-label, multicenter, phase II study. Cancer Res Treat 2018;50(2):488–94.

27. Park I, Lee SH, Lee JL. A multicenter phase II trial of axitinib in patients with recurrent or metastatic non-clear-cell renal cell carcinoma who had failed prior treatment with temsirolimus. Clin Genitourin Cancer 2018;16(5):e997–1002.

28. Negrier S, Rioux-Leclercq N, Ferlay C, et al. Axitinib in first-line for patients with metastatic papillary renal cell carcinoma: Results of the multicentre, open-label, single-arm, phase II AXIPAP trial. Eur J Cancer 2020;129:107–16. https://doi.org/10.1016/j.ejca. 2020.02.001.

29. Martínez Chanzá N, Xie W, Asim Bilen M, et al. Cabozantinib in advanced non-clear-cell renal cell carcinoma: a multicentre, retrospective, cohort study. Lancet Oncol 2019;20(4):581–90. https://doi.org/ 10.1016/S1470-2045(18)30907-0.

30. Voss MH, Molina AM, Chen Y-B, et al. Phase II trial and correlative genomic analysis of everolimus plus bevacizumab in advanced non-clear cell renal cell carcinoma. J Clin Oncol 2016;34(32):3846–53.

31. Linehan WM, Rouault TA. Molecular pathways: fumarate hydratase-deficient kidney cancer–targeting the Warburg effect in cancer. Clin Cancer Res 2013;19(13):3345–52.

32. Singer EA, Friend JC, Hawks G, et al. A phase II study of bevacizumab and erlotinib in subjects with advanced hereditary leiomyomatosis and renal cell cancer (HLRCC) or sporadic papillary renal cell cancer (RCC). J Clin Oncol 2012;30(15_suppl): TPS4680.

33. Srinivasan R, Su D, Stamatakis L, et al. Mechanism based targeted therapy for hereditary

leiomyomatosis and renal cell cancer (HLRCC) and sporadic papillary renal cell carcinoma: interim results from a phase 2 study of bevacizumab and erlotinib. Eur J Cancer 2014;50:8.

34. Choueiri TK, Plimack E, Arkenau H-T, et al. Biomarker-based phase II trial of savolitinib in patients with advanced papillary renal cell cancer. J Clin Oncol 2017;35(26):2993–3001.

35. Choueiri TK, Vaishampayan U, Rosenberg JE, et al. Phase II and biomarker study of the dual MET/VEGFR2 inhibitor foretinib in patients with papillary renal cell carcinoma. J Clin Oncol 2013;31(2):181–6.

36. Schöffski P, Wozniak A, Escudier B, et al. Crizotinib achieves long-lasting disease control in advanced papillary renal-cell carcinoma type 1 patients with MET mutations or amplification. EORTC 90101 CREATE trial. Eur J Cancer 2017;87:147–63.

37. Twardowski PW, Tangen CM, Wu X, et al. Parallel (randomized) phase II evaluation of tivantinib (ARQ197) and tivantinib in combination with erlotinib in papillary renal cell carcinoma: SWOG S1107. Kidney Cancer 2017;1(2):123–32.

38. Motzer RJ, Escudier B, McDermott DF, et al. Nivolumab versus everolimus in advanced renal-cell carcinoma. N Engl J Med 2015;373(19):1803–13.

39. Koshkin VS, Barata PC, Zhang T, et al. Clinical activity of nivolumab in patients with non-clear cell renal cell carcinoma. J Immunother Cancer 2018;6(1):9.

40. Chahoud J, Msaouel P, Campbell MT, et al. Nivolumab for the treatment of patients with metastatic non-clear cell renal cell carcinoma (nccRCC): a single-institutional experience and literature meta-analysis. Oncologist 2020;25(3):252–8.

41. McKay RR, Bossé D, Xie W, et al. The clinical activity of PD-1/PD-L1 inhibitors in metastatic non-clear cell renal cell carcinoma. Cancer Immunol Res 2018;6(7):758–65.

42. Boilève A, Carlo MI, Barthélémy P, et al. Immune checkpoint inhibitors in MITF family translocation renal cell carcinomas and genetic correlates of exceptional responders. J Immunother Cancer 2018;6(1):159.

43. Lee J-L, Ziobro M, Gafanov R, et al. KEYNOTE-427 cohort B: first-line pembrolizumab (PEMBRO) monotherapy for advanced non–clear cell renal cell carcinoma (NCC-RCC). J Clin Oncol 2019;37(15_suppl):4569.

44. McGregor BA, McKay RR, Braun DA, et al. Results of a multicenter phase II study of atezolizumab and bevacizumab for patients with metastatic renal cell carcinoma with variant histology and/or sarcomatoid features. J Clin Oncol 2019;38(1):63–70.

45. Powles T, Larkin JMG, Patel P, et al. A phase II study investigating the safety and efficacy of savolitinib and durvalumab in metastatic papillary renal cancer (CALYPSO). J Clin Oncol 2019;37(7_suppl):545.

46. Danson S, Hook J, Marshall H, et al. Are we over-treating with checkpoint inhibitors? Br J Cancer 2019;121(8):629–30.

47. McDermott DF, Huseni MA, Atkins MB, et al. Clinical activity and molecular correlates of response to atezolizumab alone or in combination with bevacizumab versus sunitinib in renal cell carcinoma. Nat Med 2018;24(6):749–57.

48. Rini BI, Huseni M, Atkins MB, et al. LBA31Molecular correlates differentiate response to atezolizumab (atezo) + bevacizumab (bev) vs sunitinib (sun): results from a phase III study (IMmotion151) in untreated metastatic renal cell carcinoma (mRCC). Ann Oncol 2018;29(suppl_8).

49. Escudier B, Molinie V, Bracarda S, et al. Open-label phase 2 trial of first-line everolimus monotherapy in patients with papillary metastatic renal cell carcinoma: RAPTOR final analysis. Eur J 2016;69:226–35.

Neoadjuvant Therapy for Locally Advanced Renal Cell Carcinoma

Mary E. Westerman, MD, Daniel D. Shapiro, MD, Christopher G. Wood, MD, Jose A. Karam, MD*

KEYWORDS

- Neoadjuvant therapy • Targeted therapy • Immune checkpoint inhibitor • Renal cell carcinoma
- Locally advanced • Nephrectomy • Partial nephrectomy

KEY POINTS

- Currently, no level 1 evidence exists to support the use of neoadjuvant therapy for locally advanced renal cell carcinoma.
- Proposed benefits of neoadjuvant therapy include tumor downsizing to facilitate resection or nephron-sparing and -shrinking renal vein thrombi.
- Multiple ongoing phase I/II trials are investigating immune checkpoint inhibitors along with combination therapy.
- Outside of a clinical trial and exceptional clinical scenarios, there is no role for routine neoadjuvant therapy use. It may have utility in patients with absolute indications for partial nephrectomy or unresectable disease.

INTRODUCTION

In 2018, there were an estimated 403,262 cases of kidney cancer diagnosed world-wide.[1] Although the incidence of early stage disease has increased, up to 40% of patients still present with locally advanced (≥cT3 and/or N1) or metastatic disease.[2] Renal cell carcinoma (RCC) is inherently chemotherapy resistant with an overall response rate (ORR) of just 5.6% to cytotoxic agents.[3] Based on randomized control trials showing improved survival compared with interferon alone, nephrectomy has been the treatment of choice for both locally advanced and metastatic disease.[4,5] Although surgical resection is the only definitive cure for RCC, recurrence rates may exceed 60% among the highest-risk patients.[6,7] However, before 2006 the available therapies were highly toxic with low efficacy and thus had little role in the perioperative setting.[8,9] After the US Food and Drug Administration approved sunitinib, a small molecule tyrosine kinase inhibitor (TKI), for cytokine-refractory metastatic RCC (mRCC) there was renewed interest in perioperative systemic therapy.[10] Subsequent trials in both the adjuvant and neoadjuvant space have been conducted, culminating in the 2018 approval of sunitinib for adjuvant therapy among high-risk patients with clear cell RCC (ccRCC).[11]

In RCC, the Von-Hippel-Lindau tumor suppressor gene is commonly mutated. This leads to persistence of hypoxia inducible factor and subsequent overtranscription of vascular endothelial growth factor (VEGF), ultimately resulting in stimulated angiogenesis.[12,13] The development of agents targeting the VEGF pathway and other pathways ushered in the targeted therapy (TT) era and new interest in preoperative therapy. Targeted therapies include TKIs (sorafenib, sunitinib, pazopanib, axitinib, cabozantinib, and lenvatinib), mammalian target of rapamycin inhibitors

Department of Urology, The University of Texas MD Anderson Cancer Center, 1515 Holcombe Boulevard, Unit 1373, Houston, TX 77030, USA
* Corresponding author.
E-mail address: JAKaram@mdanderson.org

Urol Clin N Am 47 (2020) 329–343
https://doi.org/10.1016/j.ucl.2020.04.010
0094-0143/20/© 2020 Elsevier Inc. All rights reserved.

(everolimus, temsirolimus), and bevacizumab, an anti-VEGF monoclonal antibody. To date, most published studies on presurgical therapy have used TT agents.

In 2015, nivolumab, an immune checkpoint inhibitor (ICI) targeting PD-1, was approved as second-line therapy for mRCC after demonstrating an ORR of 25% in CheckMate-025.[14] ICIs target immune cell-specific regulatory pathways such as PD-1/PD-L1, and CTLA-4, promoting antitumor immunity. In recent trials, ICIs have shown ORR of 37% to 59%, leading to both single agent and combination approvals in the metastatic setting.[15–18] In addition, with combination therapy, complete response (CR) rates have ranged from 5% to 9%.[15–18] Thus, current trials are now evaluating these agents in the perioperative setting.

Importantly, early presurgical therapy trials often contained two subsets of patients: those with no evidence of metastatic disease (M0) for whom therapy was *neoadjuvant* and those with metastatic disease (M1) for whom therapy was considered *pseudoneoadjuvant* or *presurgical*.[19] Pseudo-neoadjuvant therapy may serve as a litmus test to identify patients who may not benefit from cytoreductive nephrectomy (CN), a strategy with support from multiple phase II trials, and hypothesis-generating results from SURTIME trial and posthoc analysis of the CARMENA trial.[20–22]

METHODS

PubMed, Cochrane Central Register of Controlled Trials, and ClinicalTrials.gov were searched with keywords including "neoadjuvant, renal cell carcinoma, nephrectomy, targeted therapy, immune checkpoint inhibitors, mammalian target of rapamycin inhibitors, and tyrosine kinase inhibitors." Publications were included if they included patients with localized RCC. Articles with language other than English, editorials, and case reports were excluded.

The existing literature consists of case series, retrospective single and multiinstitution analyses, and small prospective phase I/II single arm clinical trials. Only a single prospective randomized clinical trial has been completed.[23] Objective measures used to assess tumor response to neoadjuvant therapy include Response Evaluation Criteria in Solid Tumors (RECIST) criteria and RENAL nephrometry score.[24] By RECIST, the ORR is a combination of the complete response (CR) rate and partial response (PR) rate, defined as at least a 30% decrease in the sum of diameters of target lesions.[24] Subjective assessments based on objective data include ability to resect previously unresectable disease, ability to perform partial nephrectomy, and alteration in surgical approach.

In terms of safety and tolerability, drug toxicity is recorded using the Common Terminology Criteria for Adverse Events (CTCAE) and complications using the Clavien-Dindo Classification system.[25]

RATIONALE FOR NEOADJUVANT THERAPY

Given the high recurrence rates with locally advanced disease, rationale for neoadjuvant therapy includes both improvement in oncologic outcomes (recurrence-free survival or overall survival [OS]) as well as facilitation and improving risk profile of complex resections.[26] Neoadjuvant therapy may eradicate micrometastatic disease, thus decreasing recurrence rates and improving overall survival.[21,27] Others hypothesize that with the tumor in situ, proangiogenic and/or proimmunogenic factors may enhance the efficacy of targeted therapy.[28] Likewise higher disease burden may promote systemic inflammation and greater immune system activation.[28]

Neoadjuvant therapy may facilitate the resection of surgically complex tumors, allowing unresectable tumors to become resectable and decrease the need for adjacent organ resection. For those with imperative indications for renal preservation, it may allow for an organ-sparing approach and facilitate patient recovery if minimally invasive surgery can be performed.[26,29] Finally, in the case of inferior vena cava (IVC) tumor thombi, therapy may theoretically shrink the tumor thrombus, decreasing surgical morbidity and/or reduce the need for major vascular resection.

OUTCOMES OF NEOADJUVANT THERAPY STUDIES
High-Risk Localized Renal Cell Carcinoma

To date, there are no randomized trials that evaluate the impact of neoadjuvant therapy on oncologic outcomes. In the adjuvant setting, the S-TRAC trial demonstrated a benefit of sunitinib in improving progression-free survival (PFS) but no benefit for OS.[11] Other trials in the adjuvant setting including ASSURE, PROTECT, and ATLAS have shown no benefit.[30–32] Given the limited efficacy demonstrated in the adjuvant setting with targeted therapy, a randomized neoadjuvant trial investigating survival outcomes may be difficult to conduct.[19]

Tumor Downsizing

Table 1 summarizes the reported response rates in prospective perioperative therapy trials that include locally advanced, M0 patients.

Table 1
Summary of prospective neoadjuvant clinical trials

Study, Year	N	Agent	Dose	Duration	Discontinuation Before Surgery	Inclusion Criteria	Median % Decrease in Diameter[a] (Range %) cm Decrease in Diameter	PR by RECIST	PN/RN
Hellenthal,[36] 2010	20	Sunitinib	37.5 mg PO QD	3 mo	5 d: N = 5 24 h: N = 15	≥cT1bNanyMany ccRCC M1: 20%	Mean: 11.8% (27% - +11%)	5%	8/12
Cowey,[33] 2010	30	Sorafenib	400 mg PO BID	Median: 33 d (8–59)	24–48 h	≥cT2NanyMany M1: 43%	9.6% (40% - +16%) 0.8 cm	7%	0/30
Silberstein,[37] 2010	12[b]	Sunitinib	50 mg PO QD[c]	12 wk	2 wk	cTanyNanyMany ccRCC Indication for NSS M1: 41%	Mean: 21.1% (45% - 3.2%) 1.5 cm	16%	14/0
Rini,[38] 2012	28	Sunitinib	50 mg QD	6–120 wk	≥ 7 d	cTanyNanyMany Unresectable M1: 63%	22% (100% - +13%) 1.2 cm	25%	9/4
Karam,[40] 2014	24	Axitinib	5 mg BID	12 wk	36 h	cT2-T3N0M0 ccRCC	28.3% (42.9% - 5.3%) 3.1 cm	46%	5/19
Rini,[35] 2015	25	Pazopanib	800 mg PO QD	8–16 wk	≥ 7 d	cTanyNanyM0 ccRCC Indication for NSS	26% (43% - +2%) 1.5 cm	36%	20[d]/8
Lebacle,[41] 2018	18	Axitinib	5mg PO BID[e]	8–32 wk	6 d	cT2aN0M0 ccRCC	17% (29.4% - 4.8%) 1.2 cm	22%	16/1[f]
Hatiboglu,[23,9] 2017	12	Sorafenib	400 mg PO BID vs placebo	4 wk	24 h	cT1-3N0M0	29% (61% - 4.9%) 1 cm	44% vs 0%[h]	4/5 1/2

[a] Positive numbers (increase in size) bolded.
[b] 14 kidneys, 2 patients with bilateral disease.
[c] 6 wk cycle: 4 wk on, 2 wk off.
[d] 17 patients, 3 bilateral partials (n = 20 total PN).
[e] Allowed up titration.
[f] 1 patient did not undergo surgery.
[g] RCT: 3:1 Sorafenib versus Placebo.
[h] Inferred from Fig 2, Hatiboglu et al, 2017.

In 2010, Cowey and colleagues[33] administered sorafenib to 30 patients with stage II or higher renal masses, of whom 56% had locally advanced disease (the remainder were M1). Median reduction in tumor diameter was 9.6% and only 4% had a PR based on RECIST criteria.[33] They also evaluated masses using the modified Choi criteria and found a median decrease in intratumoral enhancement of 13%, potentially representing radiographic tumor necrosis.[34]

Multiple studies, both prospective and retrospective, have evaluated the efficacy of presurgical sunitinib in a locally advanced and/or metastatic population.[23,33,35,36] Among 4 prospective series, the median decrease in tumor diameter ranged from 11.8% to 22%, with a PR rate of 7% to 37% among studies reporting RECIST criteria.[33,36–38] Importantly, none reported PD during treatment. Among retrospective series, Lane and colleagues[39] published the largest, composed of 72 patients and enriched with nonmetastatic locally advanced disease (n = 60). Treatment with sunitinib resulted in a 32% reduction in tumor area with 19% of patients experiencing a PR.[39] In addition, they reported that clear cell histology, low Fuhrman grade, and lack of lymph node disease were associated with better radiographic response.[39]

Other TKIs prospectively evaluated include pazopanib, axitinib, and sorafenib.[23,35,40,41] The only prospective randomized control trial was conducted by Hatiboglu and colleagues[23] in which 12 patients were randomized 3:1 to either sorafenib or placebo. The sorafenib arm demonstrated a median tumor reduction of 29% and 4 of 9 had a decrease in RENAL nephrometry score.[23] Rini and colleagues[35] conducted a phase II trial of pazopanib given to 25 patients with nonmetastatic disease. They reported a median tumor decrease of 26%, PR rate of 32%, and decrease in RENAL nephrometry score of 36%.[35]

Two prospective phase II trials using neoadjuvant axitinib have been published.[40,41] The first was by Karam and colleagues,[40] in which 24 patients with cT3aN0M0 disease received up to 12 weeks of neoadjuvant axitinib. They demonstrated a 28% decrease in tumor diameter with a median RENAL nephrometry score change from 11 to 10.[40] A second study was published by Lebacle and colleagues[41] in 2019. Among this cohort of patients with T2aN0M0 disease, they reported a 17% reduction in tumor size and 66% downstaging rate.[41]

Changing Unresectable to Resectable

The first published report of presurgical therapy was in 2008 by Van der Veldt and colleagues.[42]

In their retrospective report of 17 patients with mRCC given 4 weeks of sunitinib, 3 of 10 tumors initially deemed unresectable were able to be surgically removed.[42] Thomas and colleagues[26] treated 19 patients with unresectable disease with 50 mg of sunitinib daily for 4 weeks. Sixteen percent of patients had a PR by RECIST.[26] The median tumor size reduction was 24% and 21% (4/19) eventually underwent nephrectomy.[26] Likewise, Bex and colleagues[43] retrospectively identified 10 patients in whom CN was deferred due to "doubtful resectability" in the setting of metastatic disease. Three of the ten patients underwent successful CN after downsizing of the primary site and response in the metastatic sites to sunitinib.[43] Initially, all 3 patients had evidence of liver invasion, which was confirmed histologically at the time of resection—thus despite downsizing there was no downstaging.[43]

In a prospective phase II trial, Rini and colleagues[38] administered sunitinib 50 mg daily in patients with biopsy confirmed unresectable RCC. Twenty-nine patients, 66% with metastatic disease, met the definition of unresectable—large tumor (7%), bulky lymphadenopathy with vessel encasement (31%), venous thrombosis (21%), and/or proximity to vital structures(41%).[38] Thirteen patients (45%) met the primary endpoint, surgical resection, of whom 9 underwent partial nephrectomy and 4 underwent radical nephrectomy.[38] The investigators conclude that the modest decrease in tumor size (1.3 cm) may affect surgical approach in specific clinical contexts, such as partial versus radical nephrectomy in a patient with a hilar tumor and solitary kidney.[38] However, the ability to remove a large tumor with bulky nodes is not likely to be enhanced by sunitinib.[38]

In summary, a locally advanced tumor deemed unresectable in the absence of metastatic disease is rare. Although neoadjuvant therapy may decrease the tumor diameter, it is unlikely to affect surgical planning in large, bulky disease.

Converting from Radical to Partial Nephrectomy

The utility of neoadjuvant therapy to allow for partial as opposed to radical nephrectomy has also been explored. Patients with bulky bilateral tumors, locally advanced disease in a solitary kidney, or with compromised renal function have been hypothesized to benefit from nephron-sparing surgery (NSS).[37] Silberstein published a retrospective review and prospective pilot of the utility of sunitinib in this setting. Twelve patients (14 renal units), 5 with metastatic disease, who had complex tumors (collecting system abutment, hilar vessel invasion) received sunitinib and subsequently underwent successful NSS.[37] Of the 14 renal units, 3 developed urine leaks, which healed with conservative management.[37]

Lane published a retrospective review of 72 patients (78 renal units) who received presurgical sunitinib at 4 centers.[39] The indication for therapy was for bulky/central renal tumors not amenable to partial nephrectomy (PN) (60%) or patients with mRCC having a low relative volume of disease in the primary tumor (40%).[39] The median nephrometry score decreased from 10% to 9% and 63% of patients underwent PN, including 76% of nonmetastatic patients.[39]

Rini and colleagues[35] conducted a prospective phase II trial of 8 to 12 weeks of pazopanib among 25 patients with locally advanced ccRCC requiring maximal preservation of renal parenchyma. Patients were eligible if radical nephrectomy (RN) or PN would yield GFR less than 30 mL/min/1.73 m^2 and/or there was an anticipated increased risk of morbidity with PN due to high complexity (RENAL score: 10–12) or hilar tumor location.[35] The primary endpoint was completion of NSS and secondary endpoint was the amount of vascularized parenchyma that could be preserved compared with pretherapy assessment.[35] Based on surgeon assessment, partial nephrectomy was not feasible before therapy in 13/25 patients due to tumor anatomy.[35] Six of these thirteen patients ultimately underwent NSS (46%), and the amount of functional parenchyma spared increased from 107 to 173 cc.[35] For all other patients who had an imperative indication for renal preservation, the amount of parenchyma spared increased from 178 to 204 cc.[35] Five of seven patients who underwent RN required eventual dialysis as did one patient who underwent PN.[35] Among the 20 PN performed, there were 5 urine leaks (25%).[35]

McDonald and colleagues[44] conducted a multiinstitutional retrospective review comparing outcomes of patients with imperative indication for PN (n = 125) who received neoadjuvant therapy (n = 47) with those who did not (n = 78). A total of 29.8% of patients who received sunitinib experienced CTCAE grade 3 or higher toxicity.[44] They found that the low-grade 30-day complication rate was higher in the neoadjuvant group (P = .042), but there was no difference in high-grade complications (P = .73).[44] Likewise they reported no difference in positive margin rates or renal function.[44] On multivariable analysis, receipt of neoadjuvant therapy did not predict long-term renal function outcomes.[44] Thus, the investigators conclude that for complex tumors neoadjuvant

therapy before PN does not negatively affect long-term outcomes.[44]

AXIPAN was a multiinstitutional phase II trial of neoadjuvant axitinib for patients with cT2 ccRCC and normal renal function.[41] The primary endpoint was downsizing of cT2 tumors to less than 7 cm so that PN could be performed according to standard of care.[41] Patients were deemed not eligible for PN by the treating surgeon and tumor board review.[41] The primary outcome was the percentage of patients receiving PN for cT1 renal mass after no more than 6 months of therapy.[41] A total of 18 patients were enrolled, with a median tumor size of 7.6 cm and RENAL score of 11.[41] Following treatment, median tumor size decreased to 6.4 cm and RENAL score to 10.[41] Overall, 67% (12/17) of patients met the primary endpoint and of the 17 who underwent surgery, 16 had a PN.[41] Notably, 11% of patients had a positive margin and 22% had developed metastatic disease at 2-year follow-up, attributable to the high proportion of pT3a (41%) and high-grade (47%) tumors.[41]

In summary, in patients with complex tumors and imperative indication for renal preservation (solitary kidney, bilateral disease) there may be a role for neoadjuvant therapy to facilitate PN. However, surgical approach is subjective, and the literature should be interpreted carefully.[45] Karam and colleagues[45] retrospectively reviewed imaging studies following neoadjuvant axitinib treatment to determine PN feasibility pre- and posttherapy. Among 5 independent reviewers, the odds of PN feasibility markedly increased after axitinib, but they were not able to identify which patients were more likely to benefit from axitinib based on their pretreatment scans.[45] In addition, interobserver agreement was higher for moderately complex tumors as compared with more complex tumors, which is the more clinically relevant group.[45]

Downstaging Inferior Vena Cava Thrombus

In locally advanced or metastatic disease, the presence of a tumor thrombus may increase surgical risk, with the level of the tumor thrombus correlating with perioperative complication rates, which range from 12% to 47%.[46] Thus, interest in neoadjuvant therapy to decrease thrombus level and potentially decrease surgical morbidity has been explored in several series.[47–50]

The first, by Cost and colleagues,[50] described 25 patients who received targeted therapy (sunitinib = 12, other = 13) for IVC thrombus (levels II–IV). Overall, 44% had a decrease in height (median 1.5 cm decrease), 28% increase in height, and 28% stable height.[50] There was minimal change in thrombus level—84% had stable thrombi, 12% had a decrease in thrombi level, and 4% had an increase in thrombus level.[50]

Bigot and colleagues[47] reported similar findings to Cost in a series of 14 patients treated with TT (sunitinib = 11, sorafenib = 3). In this cohort, 7% (n = 1) were downstaged, 84% were stable, and 1 patient was upstaged.[47] Overall, 43% had a decrease in thrombus height (median decrease −2 cm), 43% remained stable, and 14% had an increase in thrombus length.[47] Kwon and colleagues[48] evaluated 22 patients (sunitinib = 18, sorafenib = 4) using both RECIST and Choi criteria. They reported that 40.9% of patients achieved a partial response based on Choi criteria (decrease in size of at least 10% or decrease in attenuation of at least 15%), and this was independently associated with improved overall survival.[48] Only 2 (9%) of the patients had a PR using RECIST criteria. However, the application of this study is limited in surgical populations as the investigators did not include information related to surgical tumor thrombus levels.[48]

More recently, Field and colleagues[49] published a large multiinstitutional study comparing 51 patients who underwent either primary resection (n = 34) or neoadjuvant therapy (sunitinib) followed by surgery (n = 19). In the neoadjuvant group, they report a mean reduction in thrombus length of 25% (1.3 cm).[49] Overall, 42.1% of patients had a decrease in thrombus level, whereas 52.6% had stable thrombus level, with 27.8% experiencing a PR according to RECIST.[49] Although those who received neoadjuvant treatment had significantly lower operative blood loss, there were no other differences in surgical outcomes, including surgical approach (open vs minimally invasive) between the 2 groups.[49] Although the investigators report improved cancer-specific and all-cause mortality in the neoadjuvant group (47.1% vs 10% [P = .007] and 52.9% vs 21.1% [P = .024] respectively), this was driven by the patients who were M1 at presentation.[49] On subgroup analysis of those without metastatic disease, there was no survival difference.[49]

Although neoadjuvant therapy may decrease the size of the primary tumor, presurgical targeted therapy does not seem to have the same impact on tumor thrombus. Although Field and colleagues[49] report better response than prior studies (possibly due to uniform receipt of sunitinib), there was no impact on surgical approach or outcomes. Although they demonstrated an oncologic survival benefit for presurgical therapy, this was not seen in the true neoadjuvant group.[49] Ultimately, given the lack of significant thrombus shrinkage, there is little evidence that neoadjuvant targeted therapy use

has an impact on surgical approach and thus is of limited value.

CONCERNS WITH NEOADJUVANT THERAPY

Multiple concerns related to neoadjuvant therapy have been raised, including increased wound healing complications, increased surgical complications, drug toxicity or adverse events, and risk of disease progression with surgical delay. There was significant concern regarding safety and wound healing after Jonasch and colleagues[21] reported 21% of patients treated with presurgical bevacizumab had wound dehiscence or delayed healing. However, Cowey noted no wound-related issues with sorafenib, potentially attributable to its shorter half-life.[33] Subsequently, in a 2012 trial with sunitinib, Rini also reported no wound complications.[38] Likewise, neither Karam or Rini and colleagues[35,40] noted significant wound-related issues with axitinib or pazopanib, respectively.

Chapin and colleagues[51] retrospectively compared patients with synchronous mRCC who either underwent immediate CN or received presurgical therapy followed by CN. Although no differences were found in severe or overall complications in the 12 months after surgery, patients who received presurgical therapy were significantly more likely to have delayed (>90 days) wound complications, superficial wound dehiscence, and wound infection (odds ratio 4.14, 95% confidence interval: 1.6–10.6, P = .003).[51] Harshman and colleagues[52] found that presurgical TKI use increased the incidence of intraoperative adhesions (86% vs 58%, P = .01) among 14 patients compared with matched controls, but did not affect overall complications, bleeding, or wound healing.

Complications among prospective neoadjuvant target therapy trials are outlined in **Table 2**. There is inconsistent reporting, with not all studies using the standardized Clavien-Dindo system. However, Silberstein reported 21.4% (3/14) of patients experienced a urine leak as did 25% of the patients who received pazopanib in the trial by Rini and colleagues[35,37] To date, no data evaluating the surgical safety of ICI in the neoadjuvant setting have been published.

Grade 3 or higher CTCAE drug toxicities are also shown in **Table 2**. Approximately 30% to 80% of patients experienced grade 3 or higher toxicity. However, these generally resolved with either dose reduction or drug discontinuation.[23,33,35,36,38,40,41] In addition, Karam and colleagues[40] evaluated quality of life during the neoadjuvant therapy and found that

Table 2
Summary of complications and adverse events in prospective neoadjuvant clinical trials

Study, Year	% CTCAE Grade 3 or Higher AE	Description of Adverse Events	Dose Modifications	≥ Clavien-Dindo Grade 3 Complications	Wound Complications
Hellenthal et al,[36] 2010	40%	Grade 3: 35% Neutropenia: 10% Hand-foot: 10% Pancreatitis: 15% Grade 4: 5% Hyponatremia	Interruption: 25% Dose reduction: 10%	Not formally reported	None
Cowey et al,[33] 2010	30% (Grade 3)	Grade 3 Rash, acneiform: 13.3% Hand-foot: 6.6% Fatigue: 3.3% Headache: 3.3% Hypertension: 3.3%	Dose reduction: 33%	Not formally reported	Superficial wound breakdown: 1 (POD 8)
Silberstein et al,[37] 2010	NR	NR	NR	Not formally reported *Urine leak: 21.4%*	None
Rini et al,[38] 2012	7% (Grade 4)	Grade 3/4[a] Dermatologic: 14% Mucositis: 3% Thrombocytopenia: 21% Fatigue: 10% Diarrhea: 7% Anorexia: 3% Bleeding: 3% Hypertension: 34% Neutropenia: 14% Anemia: 10%	NR	Not formally reported	None
Karam et al,[40] 2014	79% (Grade 3)	Grade 3 Hypertension: 41.7% Fatigue: 4.2% Oral mucositis: 4.2% Hand-foot syndrome: 4.2% LFT elevation: 8.3% Abdominal pain: 8.3% AKI: 4.2% Thrombocytopenia:4.2%	Discontinuation: 8.3% (11, 7 wk)	Grade 3: 8.3% Chylous ascites: 4.2% Bleeding: 4.2%	Superficial wound complication: 4.2%

(continued on next page)

Table 2
(continued)

Study, Year	% CTCAE Grade 3 or Higher AE	Description of Adverse Events	Dose Modifications	≥ Clavien-Dindo Grade 3 Complications	Wound Complications
Rini[35] 2015	64% (Grade 3)	Grade 3 Fatigue: 8% Elevated LFTs: 20% Hypertension: 36% Thrombocytopenia: 4%	NR	Grade 3: 8% Stent for urine leak: 5% Angioembolization: 5% Urine Leak: 25%	Wound infection: 8%
Lebacle et al,[41] 2018	27.7% (Grade 3)	Not provided Serious adverse event (11.1%) Impaired condition: 5.5% Polycythemia: 5.5%	Dose reduction: 5.5% Discontinuation: 16.7%	Overall: 28% *Grade 3: 16.6%* *Embolization: 5.6%* *Urine leak: 11.2%* *Grade 4: 5.6%* Suicide attempt *Grade 5: 5.6%* MI	None
Hatiboglu et al,[23] 2017	66%[b] (Grade 3)	Grade 3[c] Hand-foot syndrome: 44.4% Hypertension: 11.1% Serious adverse event: 11.1% Generalized exanthema	Dose reduction: 66% Discontinuation: 11%	Grade 5: 5.5% MI (death): placebo	None

Abbreviations: AE, adverse events; AKI, acute kidney injury; LFT, liver function test; MI, miocardial infarction; POD, postoperative day.
[a] 2 Grade 4: MI, neutropenia.
[b] Calculated based on sorafenib arm (n = 9) only.
[c] Complication detail not fully recorded.
Data from Refs.[23,33,35–38,40,41]

quality of life was significantly decreased at week 7 compared with baseline ($P = .0004$) but had returned to baseline by week 19 ($P = .3$).

Another concern with the use of neoadjuvant therapy was the risk of progressive disease (PD) among nonresponders. PD may be attributed to the documented rebound phenomenon, due to early revascularization or tumoral edema following TKI discontinuation.[53,54] Although no studies reported PD during neoadjuvant treatment, in an analysis of 66 patients who received 2 to 3 cycles of sunitinib, Powles reported that 36% of patients experienced PD during the 4-week wait before CN.[55] Similarly, they reported that 26% of patients experienced PD during a phase II trial evaluating presurgical pazopanib in the mRCC setting, again highlighting the importance of surgical timing.[56] Given that these reports are in the metastatic setting, they may not be applicable to the neoadjuvant setting.

In summary, although it seems safe to delay surgery to administer neoadjuvant therapy, most patients do experience some degree of drug toxicity, which typically resolves with dose reduction or drug discontinuation. Those who undergo partial nephrectomy may have a higher risk of urine leak, although given the small sample sizes, it is not possible to control for other confounding variables. Although there were some reports of increased wound complications related to TT, overall complication rates are equivalent. However, it remains to be seen whether this will be true with the newer ICI agents.

PREDICTING RESPONSE TO NEOADJUVANT THERAPY

Limited data exist regarding factors that predict response to neoadjuvant therapy for localized or locally advanced RCC. Investigations regarding predictors of tumor response performed in the metastatic setting have been generally extrapolated to the neoadjuvant setting; however, these findings require actual validation in the nonmetastatic setting.

Among patients treated with tyrosine kinase inhibitors, Voss et al evaluated associations between survival and mutation status of select genes of interest commonly mutated in RCC (PBRM1, STED2, KDM5C, BAP1, TP53, and TERT).[57] They demonstrated that the mutational status of BAP1, PBRM1, and TP53 were independently prognostic among patients with advanced or mRCC treated with 1st line TKIs.[57] Beuselinck et al previously performed ccRCC transcriptome analysis and identified four ccRCC subtypes (ccrcc1-4) with varying responses to sunitinib

therapy.[58] Lower response rates and shorter PFS/OS were identified among ccrcc1 and ccrcc4 tumors compared to ccrcc2 and ccrcc3 tumors.[58]

The development of checkpoint inhibitors has led to a significant effort to identify biomarkers for tumor response; however, no validated predictive markers currently exist. The degree of PD-L1 expression has been evaluated with differing results. The Javelin Renal 101 trial demonstrated improved PFS among mRCC patients receiving axitinib with avelumab compared with sunitinib in both the PD-L1 positive tumors as well as in the overall population.[18] Similarly, CheckMate 214 demonstrated that among patients with mRCC, PD-L1 expression greater than or equal to 1% had an objective response rate of 58% compared with the objective response rate for PD-L1 expression less than 1% of 37% after exposure to nivolumab/ipilimumab.[17] This trial also demonstrated that OS and PFS was improved for nivolumab/ipilimumab compared with sunitinib regardless of PD-L1 expression level.[17] Tumor mutational burden and characterization of the tumor infiltrating lymphocytes have also been evaluated as potential predictors of response to checkpoint inhibitors. Overall, these biomarkers are limited as a predictive biomarker given the heterogeneity of expression in the primary tumor and unclear cutoffs that define positivity.[59] Future investigations will require not only identifying effective neoadjuvant therapies but also biomarkers that may predict success.

OUR CURRENT PRACTICE

At our center, we only use neoadjuvant therapy (i.e. limited to non-metastatic patients) in few selected situations. First: in the setting of a neoadjuvant clinical trial (the most common scenario). Second: when a patient has a solitary kidney, with a large tumor that is not felt to be amenable to partial nephrectomy safely (either from an oncologic perspective, or from a functional renal remnant perspective). Third: when a patient has a large tumor with local invasion into adjacent organs (cT4) in the setting of sarcomatoid RCC. Fourth: in the setting of "unresectable" disease, which is the least common scenario. In all these situation, we always consult our Interventional Radiology colleagues to perform percutaneous image-guided core biopsies to establish the histologic subtype and diagnosis, and to obtain specimens for research when indicated.

FUTURE DIRECTIONS

With the approval of ICI for use in mRCC, there has been interest in evaluating these drugs in the

Table 3
Summary of ongoing clinical trials of neoadjuvant therapy in locally advanced renal cell carcinoma

NCT Trial #	Agent	Phase	N	Dose	Duration (Weeks)	Inclusion[a]	Primary Outcome(s)	Status[b]	Est. Completion
Neoadjuvant Phase I/II trials for locally advanced renal cell carcinoma									
NCT01361113[64]	Pazopanib	II	21	800 mg QD	8	• T2a-T4NanyM0	ORR → 38.1%	Completed	1/2015
NCT02575222[68]	Nivolumab	I	30	3mg/kg q2W	6	• T2a-T4NanyM0 • TanyN1M0	Safety[c]	Active, not recruiting	6/2020
NCT02595918[67]	Nivolumab	I	29	IV q2W	8	• Resectable, high risk M0 • M1 undergoing CN or meta-stasectomy	Feasibility to receive at least 3 doses without significant surgical delay[d]	Recruiting	4/2021
NCT02762006[66]	Durvalumab & Tremelimumab	Ib	45	Durvalumab x 1 Or Durvalumab & Tremelimumab x 1[e]		• T2b-4 NanyM0 • TanyN1M0 • Any histology	Dose limiting toxicity	Active, not recruiting	11/2020
NCT04028245[61] SPARC-1	Spartalizumab & Canakinumab	I	14	Spartalizumab: 300 mg q4w x 2 doses Canakinumab: 400 mg IV q4w x 2 doses	8	• T2-T4N0M0 • TanyN1M0	% who proceed to RN within 6 wks	Recruiting	12/2021
NCT03438708[65] PADRES	Axitinib	II	50	5mg BID[f]	8-10	• TanyNanyM0 with imperative indication for NSS	• % reduction of longest diameter in mm • ORR • Δ in R.E.N.A.L. score • PN feasibility	Unknown[g]	2/2020
NCT04022343[62]	Cabozantinib	II	17	60 mg QD[h]	12	• T3-T4NanyM0 • TanyN1M0 • Unresectable	ORR	Recruiting	08/2023

NCT	Therapy	Phase	N	Dose		Inclusion	Primary endpoint	Status	Completion
NCT04118885[69]	Axitinib & Toripalimab	II	30	Axitinib: 5 mg BID Toripalimab: 3 mg/kg q3w x3	12	• T2-T3N0M0	ORR	Open, not recruiting	3/2026
NCT03341845[71] NeoAvAx	Axitinib & Avelumab	II	40	Axitinib: 5 mg BID Avelumab: 10 mg/kg q2W	12	• Int/high risk locally advanced RCC	Partial remission	Recruiting	1/2025
NCT03680521[70]	Sitravatinib & Nivolumab	II	25	Sitravatinib QD x 2 wk then with nivolumab 240 mg IV q2W	6–8	• Locally advanced RCC	ORR	Recruiting	4/2020
Thrombus Trials									
NCT02473536[63]	SABR	I/II	30	8Gy/5Frac or 12 Gy/3Frac		• ≥ level II IVC tumor thrombus, surgically resectable • Any Histology	Phase 1: safety[i] Phase 2: RFS	Active, not recruiting	12/2024
NCT03494816[60] NAXIVA	Axitinib	II	20	5mg BID[j]	8	• T3a-NanyMany	Improvement in Mayo Classification	Recruiting	6/2020

a Limited to ccRCC unless otherwise specified.
b As of 06/2020.
c Any CTCAE adverse event from initial dose through 100 d post-surgery.
d Significant surgical delay defined as ≥112 d after first nivolumab dose.
e Both arms include multiple cohorts with varying adjuvant dosages.
f Allows for dose escalation as tolerated.
g Recruiting as of 12/2019; unknown as of 06/2020.
h Two dose reductions allowed.
i 90 d Grade 4 to 5 adverse events attributable to SABR.
j Allows for dose escalation.

neoadjuvant setting with or without the addition of TKIs. **Table 3** lists the active clinical trials as of October, 2019. Currently, there are 8 open trials investigating neoadjuvant therapy in nonmetastatic RCC and 2 that are closed and awaiting results.[60–71] One, NCT01361113, which evaluated Pazopanib in a phase II trial among localized ccRCC, recently reported an ORR of 38.1%.[64] The primary endpoint for most of the phase II trials is ORR alone, with the exception of PADRES (NCT03438708).[65] This multicenter study of neoadjuvant axitinib is limited to patients with complex renal masses and imperative indication for nephron preservation.[65] In addition to ORR, the study aims include ability to perform partial nephrectomy and avoidance of renal replacement therapy.[65] In addition, there are also 2 open evaluating neoadjuvant therapy for IVC thrombi.[60,63] NCT02473536 is a combined phase I/II trial of stereotactic ablative body radiation for greater than or equal to level 2 tumor thrombi, whereas NAXIVA (NCT03494816) is evaluating the response of tumor thrombi to axitinib.[60,63]

SUMMARY

There is limited data to support the use of neoadjuvant therapy outside of a clinical trial. Neoadjuvant TT for tumor downsizing alone is of limited benefit for bulky, unresectable tumors and has shown minimal utility in patients with IVC thrombi. In select patients, neoadjuvant therapy may facilitate NSS, but the definitions of "unresectable" or "not amenable to PN" are subjective. A multidisciplinary discussion should be undertaken when considering neoadjuvant therapy, particularly in experienced centers. Future trials will determine whether there is a role for ICI in the neoadjuvant setting.

REFERENCES

1. Bray F, Ferlay J, Soerjomataram I, et al. Global cancer statistics 2018: GLOBOCAN estimates of incidence and mortality worldwide for 36 cancers in 185 countries. CA Cancer J Clin 2018;68(6): 394–424.
2. Kane CJ, Mallin K, Ritchey J, et al. Renal cell cancer stage migration: analysis of the National Cancer Data Base. Cancer 2008;113(1):78–83.
3. Yagoda A, Petrylak D, Thompson S. Cytotoxic chemotherapy for advanced renal cell carcinoma. Urol Clin North Am 1993;20(2):303–21.
4. Flanigan RC, Salmon SE, Blumenstein BA, et al. Nephrectomy followed by interferon alfa-2b compared with interferon alfa-2b alone for metastatic renal-cell cancer. N Engl J Med 2001;345(23):1655–9.
5. Mickisch GH, Garin A, van Poppel H, et al. Radical nephrectomy plus interferon-alfa-based immunotherapy compared with interferon alfa alone in metastatic renal-cell carcinoma: a randomised trial. Lancet 2001;358(9286):966–70.
6. Leibovich BC, Blute ML, Cheville JC, et al. Prediction of progression after radical nephrectomy for patients with clear cell renal cell carcinoma: a stratification tool for prospective clinical trials. Cancer 2003; 97(7):1663–71.
7. Zisman A, Pantuck AJ, Wieder J, et al. Risk group assessment and clinical outcome algorithm to predict the natural history of patients with surgically resected renal cell carcinoma. J Clin Oncol 2002; 20(23):4559–66.
8. Negrier S, Escudier B, Lasset C, et al. Recombinant human interleukin-2, recombinant human interferon alfa-2a, or both in metastatic renal-cell carcinoma. Groupe Français d'Immunothérapie. N Engl J Med 1998;338(18):1272–8.
9. Motzer RJ, Rini BI, Bukowski RM, et al. Sunitinib in patients with metastatic renal cell carcinoma. JAMA 2006;295(21):2516–24.
10. Tobert CM, Uzzo RG, Wood CG, et al. Adjuvant and neoadjuvant therapy for renal cell carcinoma: a survey of the Society of Urologic Oncology. Urol Oncol 2013;31(7):1316–20.
11. Ravaud A, Motzer RJ, Pandha HS, et al. Adjuvant Sunitinib in High-Risk Renal-Cell Carcinoma after Nephrectomy. N Engl J Med 2016;375(23):2246–54.
12. Rini BI, Atkins MB. Resistance to targeted therapy in renal-cell carcinoma. Lancet Oncol 2009;10(10): 992–1000.
13. Rini BI. Vascular endothelial growth factor-targeted therapy in metastatic renal cell carcinoma. Cancer 2009;115(10 Suppl):2306–12.
14. Motzer RJ, Escudier B, McDermott DF, et al. Nivolumab versus Everolimus in Advanced Renal-Cell Carcinoma. N Engl J Med 2015;373(19):1803–13.
15. Rini BI, Powles T, Atkins MB, et al. Atezolizumab plus bevacizumab versus sunitinib in patients with previously untreated metastatic renal cell carcinoma (IMmotion151): a multicentre, open-label, phase 3, randomised controlled trial. Lancet 2019; 393(10189):2404–15.
16. Rini BI, Plimack ER, Stus V, et al. Pembrolizumab plus Axitinib versus Sunitinib for Advanced Renal-Cell Carcinoma. N Engl J Med 2019;380(12): 1116–27.
17. Motzer RJ, Tannir NM, McDermott DF, et al. Nivolumab plus Ipilimumab versus sunitinib in advanced renal-cell carcinoma. N Engl J Med 2018;378(14): 1277–90.
18. Motzer RJ, Penkov K, Haanen J, et al. Avelumab plus axitinib versus sunitinib for advanced renal-cell carcinoma. N Engl J Med 2019;380(12): 1103–15.

19. Bex A, Powles T, Karam JA. Role of targeted therapy in combination with surgery in renal cell carcinoma. Int J Urol 2016;23(1):5–12.

20. Mejean A, Thezenas S, Chevreau C, et al. Cytoreductive nephrectomy (CN) in metastatic renal cancer (mRCC): Update on Carmena trial with focus on intermediate IMDC-risk population. J Clin Oncol 2019;37(suppl) [abstract: 4508].

21. Jonasch E, Wood CG, Matin SF, et al. Phase II presurgical feasibility study of bevacizumab in untreated patients with metastatic renal cell carcinoma. J Clin Oncol 2009;27(25):4076–81.

22. Mejean A, Ravaud A, Thezenas S, et al. Sunitinib alone or after nephrectomy in metastatic renal-cell carcinoma. N Engl J Med 2018;379(5):417–27.

23. Hatiboglu G, Hohenfellner M, Arslan A, et al. Effective downsizing but enhanced intratumoral heterogeneity following neoadjuvant sorafenib in patients with non-metastatic renal cell carcinoma. Langenbecks Arch Surg 2017;402(4):637–44.

24. Eisenhauer EA, Therasse P, Bogaerts J, et al. New response evaluation criteria in solid tumours: revised RECIST guideline (version 1.1). Eur J Cancer 2009; 45(2):228–47.

25. Clavien PA, Barkun J, de Oliveira ML, et al. The Clavien-Dindo classification of surgical complications: five-year experience. Ann Surg 2009;250(2): 187–96.

26. Thomas AA, Rini BI, Lane BR, et al. Response of the primary tumor to neoadjuvant sunitinib in patients with advanced renal cell carcinoma. J Urol 2009; 181(2):518–23 [discussion: 523].

27. Timsit MO, Albiges L, Méjean A, et al. Neoadjuvant treatment in advanced renal cell carcinoma: current situation and future perspectives. Expert Rev Anticancer Ther 2012;12(12):1559–69.

28. Gleeson JP, Motzer RJ, Lee CH. The current role for adjuvant and neoadjuvant therapy in renal cell cancer. Curr Opin Urol 2019;29(6):636–42.

29. Posadas EM, Figlin RA. Kidney cancer: progress and controversies in neoadjuvant therapy. Nat Rev Urol 2014;11(5):254–5.

30. Gross-Goupil M, Kwon TG, Eto M, et al. Axitinib versus placebo as an adjuvant treatment of renal cell carcinoma: results from the phase III, randomized ATLAS trial. Ann Oncol 2018;29(12): 2371–8.

31. Motzer RJ, Haas NB, Donskov F, et al. Randomized Phase III trial of adjuvant pazopanib versus placebo after nephrectomy in patients with localized or locally advanced renal cell carcinoma. J Clin Oncol 2017;35(35):3916–23.

32. Haas NB, Manola J, Uzzo RG, et al. Adjuvant sunitinib or sorafenib for high-risk, non-metastatic renal-cell carcinoma (ECOG-ACRIN E2805): a double-blind, placebo-controlled, randomised, phase 3 trial. Lancet 2016;387(10032):2008–16.

33. Cowey CL, Amin C, Pruthi RS, et al. Neoadjuvant clinical trial with sorafenib for patients with stage II or higher renal cell carcinoma. J Clin Oncol 2010; 28(9):1502–7.

34. Cowey CL, Fielding JR, Rathmell WK. The loss of radiographic enhancement in primary renal cell carcinoma tumors following multitargeted receptor tyrosine kinase therapy is an additional indicator of response. Urology 2010;75(5):1108–13.e1.

35. Rini BI, Plimack ER, Takagi T, et al. A phase II study of pazopanib in patients with localized renal cell carcinoma to optimize preservation of renal parenchyma. J Urol 2015;194(2):297–303.

36. Hellenthal NJ, Underwood W, Penentrante R, et al. Prospective clinical trial of preoperative sunitinib in patients with renal cell carcinoma. J Urol 2010; 184(3):859–64.

37. Silberstein JL, Millard F, Mehrazin R, et al. Feasibility and efficacy of neoadjuvant sunitinib before nephron-sparing surgery. BJU Int 2010;106(9): 1270–6.

38. Rini BI, Garcia J, Elson P, et al. The effect of sunitinib on primary renal cell carcinoma and facilitation of subsequent surgery. J Urol 2012;187(5): 1548–54.

39. Lane BR, Derweesh IH, Kim HL, et al. Presurgical sunitinib reduces tumor size and may facilitate partial nephrectomy in patients with renal cell carcinoma. Urol Oncol 2015;33(3):112.e15-21.

40. Karam JA, Devine CE, Urbauer DL, et al. Phase 2 trial of neoadjuvant axitinib in patients with locally advanced nonmetastatic clear cell renal cell carcinoma. Eur Urol 2014;66(5):874–80.

41. Lebacle C, Bensalah K, Bernhard JC, et al. Evaluation of axitinib to downstage cT2a renal tumours and allow partial nephrectomy: a phase II study. BJU Int 2019;123(5):804–10.

42. van der Veldt AA, Meijerink MR, van den Eertwegh AJ, et al. Sunitinib for treatment of advanced renal cell cancer: primary tumor response. Clin Cancer Res 2008;14(8):2431–6.

43. Bex A, van der Veldt AA, Blank C, et al. Neoadjuvant sunitinib for surgically complex advanced renal cell cancer of doubtful resectability: initial experience with downsizing to reconsider cytoreductive surgery. World J Urol 2009;27(4):533–9.

44. McDonald ML, Lane BR, Jimenez J, et al. Renal Functional Outcome of Partial Nephrectomy for Complex R.E.N.A.L. score tumors with or without neoadjuvant sunitinib: a multicenter analysis. Clin Genitourin Cancer 2018;16(2):e289–95.

45. Karam JA, Devine CE, Fellman BM, et al. Variability of inter-observer agreement on feasibility of partial nephrectomy before and after neoadjuvant axitinib for locally advanced renal cell carcinoma (RCC): independent analysis from a phase II trial. BJU Int 2016;117(4):629–35.

46. Karnes RJ, Blute ML. Surgery insight: management of renal cell carcinoma with associated inferior vena cava thrombus. Nat Clin Pract Urol 2008;5(6): 329–39.

47. Bigot P, Fardoun T, Bernhard JC, et al. Neoadjuvant targeted molecular therapies in patients undergoing nephrectomy and inferior vena cava thrombectomy: is it useful? World J Urol 2014;32(1):109–14.

48. Kwon T, Lee JL, Kim JK, et al. The Choi response criteria for inferior vena cava tumor thrombus in renal cell carcinoma treated with targeted therapy. J Cancer Res Clin Oncol 2014;140(10):1751–8.

49. Field CA, Cotta BH, Jimenez J, et al. Neoadjuvant sunitinib decreases inferior vena caval thrombus size and is associated with improved oncologic outcomes: a multicenter comparative analysis. Clin Genitourin Cancer 2019;17(3): e505–12.

50. Cost NG, Delacroix SE, Sleeper JP, et al. The impact of targeted molecular therapies on the level of renal cell carcinoma vena caval tumor thrombus. Eur Urol 2011;59(6):912–8.

51. Chapin BF, Delacroix SE Jr, Culp SH, et al. Safety of presurgical targeted therapy in the setting of metastatic renal cell carcinoma. Eur Urol 2011;60(5): 964–71.

52. Harshman LC, Yu RJ, Allen GI, et al. Surgical outcomes and complications associated with presurgical tyrosine kinase inhibition for advanced renal cell carcinoma (RCC). Urol Oncol 2013;31(3): 379–85.

53. Mancuso MR, Davis R, Norberg SM, et al. Rapid vascular regrowth in tumors after reversal of VEGF inhibition. J Clin Invest 2006;116(10):2610–21.

54. Jain RK, Tong RT, Munn LL. Effect of vascular normalization by antiangiogenic therapy on interstitial hypertension, peritumor edema, and lymphatic metastasis: insights from a mathematical model. Cancer Res 2007;67(6):2729–35.

55. Powles T, Blank C, Chowdhury S, et al. The outcome of patients treated with sunitinib prior to planned nephrectomy in metastatic clear cell renal cancer. Eur Urol 2011;60(3):448–54.

56. Powles T, Kayani I, Sharpe K, et al. A prospective evaluation of VEGF-targeted treatment cessation in metastatic clear cell renal cancer. Ann Oncol 2013; 24(8):2098–103.

57. Voss MH, Reising A, Cheng Y, et al. Genomically annotated risk model for advanced renal-cell carcinoma: a retrospective cohort study. Lancet Oncol 2018;19(12):1688–98.

58. Beuselinck B, Job S, Becht E, et al. Molecular subtypes of clear cell renal cell carcinoma are associated with sunitinib response in the metastatic setting. Clin Cancer Res. 2015;21(6):1329–39.

59. Dudani S, Savard MF, Heng DYC. An Update on Predictive Biomarkers in Metastatic Renal Cell Carcinoma. Eur Urol Focus 2020;6(1):34–6.

60. ClinicalTrials.gov. NCT03494816, study of axitinib for reducing extent of venous tumour thrombus in renal cancer with venous invasion. Bethesda, MD: National Library of Medicine (US); 2018. Available at: https://ClinicalTrials.gov/show/NCT03494816. Accessed December 10, 2019.

61. ClinicalTrials.gov. NCT04022343, neoadjuvant cabozantinib in treating patients with locally advanced kidney cancer. Bethesda, MD: National Library of Medicine (US); 2019. Available at: https://clinicaltrials.gov/ct2/show/NCT04022343. Accessed December 10, 2019.

62. ClinicalTrials.gov. NCT04028245, A study of combination spartalizumab and canakinumab in patients with localized clear cell renal cell carcinoma (SPARC-1). Bethesda, MD: National Library of Medicine (US); 2019. Available at: https://clinicaltrials.gov/ct2/show/NCT04028245. Accessed December 10, 2019.

63. ClinicalTrials.gov. NCT02473536, neo-adjuvant SABR for IVC tumor thrombus in newly diagnosed RCC. Bethesda, MD: National Library of Medicine (US); 2015. Available at: https://clinicaltrials.gov/ct2/show/NCT02473536. Accessed December 10, 2019.

64. ClinicalTrials.gov. NCT01361113, neoadjuvant pazopanib in renal cell carcinoma. Bethesda, MD: National Library of Medicine (US); 2011. Available at: https://clinicaltrials.gov/ct2/show/NCT01361113. Accessed December 10, 2019.

65. ClinicalTrials.gov. NCT03438708, Prior Axitinib as a Determinant of Outcome of Renal Surgery (PADRES). 2018. Available at: https://clinicaltrials.gov/ct2/show/NCT03438708. Accessed December 10, 2019.

66. ClinicalTrials.gov. NCT02762006, neoadjuvant MEDI 4736 +/- tremelimumab in locally advanced renal cell carcinoma. Bethesda, MD: National Library of Medicine (US); 2016. Available at: https://clinicaltrials.gov/ct2/show/NCT02762006. Accessed December 10, 2019.

67. ClinicalTrials.gov. NCT02595918, nivolumab in treating patients with high-risk kidney cancer before surgery. Bethesda, MD: National Library of Medicine (US); 2015. Available at: https://clinicaltrials.gov/ct2/show/NCT02595918. Accessed December 10, 2019.

68. ClinicalTrials.gov. NCT02575222, study of neoadjuvant nivolumab in patients with non-metastatic stage II-IV clear cell renal cell carcinoma. Bethesda, MD: National Library of Medicine (US); 2015. Available at: https://clinicaltrials.gov/ct2/show/NCT02575222. Accessed December 10, 2019.

69. ClinicalTrials.gov. NCT04118855, toripalimab combined with axitinib as neoadjuvant therapy in patients with non-metastatic locally advanced nonmetastatic clear cell renal cell carcinoma. Bethesda, MD: National Library of Medicine (US); 2019. Available at: https://clinicaltrials.gov/ct2/show/NCT04118855. Accessed December 10, 2019.

70. ClinicalTrials.gov. NCT03680521, neoadjuvant sitravatinib in combination with nivolumab in patients with clear cell renal cell carcinoma. Bethesda, MD: National Library of Medicine (US); 2018. Available at: https://clinicaltrials.gov/ct2/show/NCT03680521. Accessed December 10, 2019.

71. ClinicalTrials.gov. NCT03341845, neoadjuvant AXITINIB and AVELUMAB for patients with localized clear-cell RCC. Bethesda, MD: National Library of Medicine (US); 2017. Available at: https://clinicaltrials.gov/ct2/show/NCT03341845. Accessed December 10, 2019.

Adjuvant Therapy for Localized High-Risk Renal Cell Carcinoma

Erika Wood, MD, MPH[a],[1], Nicholas Donin, MD[b],[2], Brian Shuch, MD[c],*

KEYWORDS

- Carcinoma • Renal cell • Chemotherapy • Adjuvant • Recurrence • Molecular targeted therapy
- Immunotherapy

KEY POINTS

- Recurrence risk following nephrectomy for kidney cancer varies widely based on disease biology, and surveillance algorithms are designed to intensify surveillance for the highest-risk individuals.
- Targeted therapy with anti–vascular endothelial growth factor receptor agents advanced the management of metastatic disease but has proved to be disappointing in the adjuvant setting, with no agents showing an improvement in overall survival.
- Several immunotherapy-based adjuvant therapy protocols are ongoing and hold promise for a future adjuvant therapy.

INTRODUCTION

Early detection has led to stage migration toward smaller and more localized forms of kidney cancer, and many individuals experience outstanding outcomes. However, approximately 10% of individuals present with stage 3 disease[1] and up to 40% of small tumors have adverse pathologic characteristics found at surgery.[2] For these high-risk patients, despite removal of all visible disease, approximately 50% recur within 6 years.[3–7]

As in many solid tumors, there is interest in providing high-risk patients with an effective adjuvant therapy that could decrease the likelihood of disease recurrence and ultimately translate into improved overall survival (OS). Numerous adjuvant therapy trials for high-risk renal cell carcinoma (RCC) have been undertaken to evaluate a wide range of agents. However, only a single trial thus far, the S-TRAC trial has shown a disease-free survival (DFS) benefit.[4] Given the potential toxicities of sunitinib, the lack of an OS benefit, and the discordance of S-TRAC's findings with other adjuvant trials, most clinicians have not changed their current practice patterns and the National Comprehensive Cancer Network (NCCN) guidelines still endorse clinical trial as the preferred option.[8] This article reviews the concepts and clinical data pertaining to adjuvant therapy for localized, high-risk RCC.

PATTERNS OF RECURRENCE, RISK FACTORS, AND RISK STRATIFICATION

Between 20% and 40% of all patients with localized kidney cancer experience a recurrence following surgery, with nearly 50% of the highest-risk patients recurring within 6 years.[3,4,7] Most recurrences occur

[a] Department of Urology, David Geffen School of Medicine at UCLA, Los Angeles, CA, USA; [b] Division of Urologic Oncology, Department of Urology, David Geffen School of Medicine at UCLA, Los Angeles, CA, USA; [c] Kidney Cancer Program, Division of Urologic Oncology, Department of Urology, David Geffen School of Medicine at UCLA, Los Angeles, CA, USA
[1] Present address: 300 Jules Stein Plaza, Wasserman Building 3rd Floor, Los Angeles, CA 90095.
[2] Present address: 2625 Alameda West Suite 310, Burbank, CA 91505.
* Corresponding author. 300 Jules Stein Plaza, Wasserman Building 3rd Floor, Los Angeles, CA 90095.
E-mail address: BShuch@mednet.ucla.edu

Urol Clin N Am 47 (2020) 345–358
https://doi.org/10.1016/j.ucl.2020.04.007

within the first 3 years of complete surgical resection; however, many occur even after 10 years following surgery.[9,10] The most common systemic sites of recurrence are the lung (64%), liver (11%), bone (15%), regional lymph nodes (9%), and the renal fossa (9%).[11] Rates of local recurrence are 1% to 6% following partial nephrectomy and 1% to 3% following radical nephrectomy, with or without systemic recurrences.[9,12]

Risk factors for recurrence include nuclear tumor grade (including Fuhrman), tumor stage, nodal involvement, microvascular invasion, necrosis, margin status, and high-risk features such as sarcomatoid or rhabdoid differentiation.[13] Specific histologic subtypes such as collecting duct, medullary, and clear cell kidney cancer may have the highest risk of dissemination.[13,14] Various series have attempted to show that histology is an independent predictor of outcome; however, all forms of renal cancer can behave aggressively.[14–16]

Risk stratification is critical for identifying a population at highest risk for recurrence, and several staging systems exist for the prediction of DFS. Most rely heavily on surgical pathologic data, such as pathologic T stage, tumor size, nuclear (Fuhrman) grade, and presence of necrosis, although a presurgical nomogram exists as well (**Table 1**).[17–21] Because these nomograms use slightly different criteria, the calculated risk of recurrence varies between them. In general, the more complex a model is, the more difficult it is to use because several histologic features may not be uniformly reported on from the surgical specimens.[22] Even among adjuvant trial patients with the highest risk, many of these nomograms still perform poorly.

Attempts have been made to move beyond traditional clinical and pathologic criteria and incorporate somatic genetic information to create more accurate prognostic models in the high-risk patient population. This information has included protein expression[23] and gene expression scores. A molecular classification system, although promising, would increase the cost and complexity of identifying patients at highest risk. Before widespread adoption, it will be important to understand whether they add incremental value justifying their use.

CONCEPTS UNDERLYING ADJUVANT THERAPY

The goal of adjuvant drug therapy is to provide additional therapy following treatment of the primary tumor in order to reduce the risk of disease recurrence and death by eliminating residual micrometastatic disease that is destined to recur.

Adjuvant treatment differs from salvage therapy in that treatment is administered based on a perceived risk of disease recurrence, but before any definitive evidence of disease recurrence. Adjuvant therapy has been shown to be a successful therapeutic strategy in various solid tumor types, including cancers of the breast, testis, ureter, ovary, and melanoma. For cancers with a serum biomarker (eg, prostate-specific antigen), detection at this level may be a useful surrogate for residual disease burden; however, such a marker does not exist in RCC. As such, clinicians must rely on prognostic models to help identify patients in whom micrometastatic disease is likely to be present.

Successful development of a therapeutic adjuvant agent must overcome the following challenges:

1. Candidate adjuvant agents must be identified. Inferring that agents successful in metastatic disease will be effective in the adjuvant setting likely depends on the mechanism of action. For example, vascular endothelial growth factor (VEGF)–targeting agents, which inhibit angiogenesis, may not function well as inhibitors of micrometastatic disease, whose biology may be less reliant on angiogenesis and nonlethal pathway inhibition.[24,25]
2. Inclusion criteria must allow for robust trial enrollment in a reasonable time frame while ensuring patients have enough risk to benefit from adjuvant therapy.
3. There must be enough power to detect a small but modest benefit. Inclusion of lower-risk patients with fewer events may limit the power to detect a smaller, but meaningful, benefit.
4. Side effect profile of any adjuvant agent must be sufficiently acceptable to justify treatment in asymptomatic patients.
5. Relevant end points must be determined. DFS has been shown to be a useful surrogate of OS in some diseases, and is an US Food and Drug Administration (FDA)–sanctioned end point in colorectal cancer and melanoma.[26,27] Although used as the primary end point in adjuvant RCC trials, some investigators have called into question whether DFS is an appropriate surrogate for OS.[28,29] There are various advantages and disadvantages to these end points in the adjuvant setting (**Table 2**).
6. The median DFS in recent adjuvant clinical trials is more than 6 years, making trials long and expensive.[3–5] With OS in the setting of metastatic disease now greater than 3 years, showing an OS difference may require a study to be open for longer than 5 years.

Table 1
Kidney cancer prognostic systems

System	Study	T Stage	N Stage	M Stage	Tumor Size	Grade	Necrosis	Histology	ECOG	MVI	Clinical Symptoms	Gender
UISS	Zisman et al,[17] 2002	1997 T stage	X	X	—	—	—	—	X	—	—	—
SSIGN	Frank et al,[18] 2002	2002 T stage	X	X	(< or ≥5 cm)	X	X	—	—	—	—	—
Leibovich	Leibovich et al,[19] 2003	2002 T-stage	X	—	(0 or >10 cm)	X	X	—	—	—	—	—
MSKCC	Kattan et al,[20] 2001	1997 T stage	—	—	Continuous	X	X	Clear cell, papillary, chromophobe	—	X	X	—
Raj[a]	Raj et al,[21] 2008	—	X	X	Continuous	—	X	—	—	—	X	X

Abbreviations: ECOG, Eastern Cooperative Group performance status; MSKCC, Memorial Sloan Kettering Cancer Center; MVI, microvascular invasion; SSIGN, stage, size, grade, and necrosis; UISS, University of California, Los Angeles, integrated staging system.
[a] Used prenephrectomy, thus N status, tumor size, and necrosis based on imaging; all others used postnephrectomy and use pathologic data.

Table 2
Comparative advantages and disadvantages of disease-free survival and overall survival as adjuvant trial end points

	Advantages	Disadvantages
DFS	• Quicker to obtain • Reliable (when central, blinded review determines recurrence)	• Unblinded investigator determination of recurrence subject to bias • Heterogeneity of imaging modalities (± contrast), detection bias possible • May not correlate with OS
OS	• Most relevant outcome for patients and physicians • Easy/reliable to collect and interpret	• May be prohibitively long to reach median survival (10–15 y), preventing expedient trial completion • Patients may lose contact after routine surveillance ends, leading to uncaptured events

ADJUVANT TRIALS OF CLASSIC IMMUNOTHERAPY AGENTS

The poor response of RCC to conventional chemotherapy, radiation, or hormone therapy, along with the discovery of the immune sensitivity of kidney cancer, led to the immunotherapy/cytokine era for advanced and metastatic RCC in the 1980s to 2000s.[30] Cytokine therapy with interferon alfa (IFN-α) and high-dose interleukin-2 (HD IL-2) offered patients with advanced disease at least some hope of a response despite a poor prognosis. Response rates for HD IL-2 in patients with metastatic RCC were 12% to 15%, with a small proportion having complete and durable response (5%–6%).[31–33] The burden of toxicity with HD IL-2, although high, was offset with the chance of a durable cure because more than 80% of complete responders had no evidence of disease at 10 years without additional treatment.[31,34] These impressive responses led HD IL-2 to become the first FDA-approved therapy for RCC. HD IL-2 remained an option at some academic centers in the targeted therapy era for highly select patients (younger, healthier, low metastatic burden); however, with impressive responses with new agents, the role of IL-2 has further diminished.[33]

Cytokines have been explored in the adjuvant setting for high-risk individuals. In a randomized study of 247 postnephrectomy patients, IFN-α2b made no difference in the rate of metastases or OS compared with controls.[35] Messing and colleagues[36] randomized 283 patients with completely resected T3 to T4a and/or node-positive disease to IFN-α or observation. There was no benefit with therapy and perhaps a worse median survival in the treatment arm (5.1 years vs 7.4 years, $P = .09$). Similarly, there was hope

for adjuvant HD IL-2 as an adjuvant therapy. The toxicity was high but expected (88% with grade 3/4 toxicity); however, efficacy was poor, with the study being closed at the interim analysis after enrolling 69 patients.[37]

Vaccines were commonly administered in conjunction with cytokines in the 1990s to improve efficacy in the metastatic setting, and were also evaluated in the adjuvant setting. German investigators randomized patients undergoing nephrectomy to 6 monthly intradermal injections of an autologous tumor vaccine versus surveillance.[38] In total, 379 patients were evaluable on the intent-to-treat analysis and a benefit was noted in progression-free survival favoring the vaccine group (hazard ratio [HR], 1.59; $P = .0204$). However, concerns about loss of patients after randomization and the absence of survival benefit prevented this therapy from becoming established as a new treatment standard. Another phase III randomized trial evaluating a different patient-derived vaccine, vitespen, was studied in 818 patients and showed no recurrence-free survival (RFS) benefit.[39] A subgroup analysis suggested some benefit in patients with intermediate-risk features, leading this agent to be approved in Russia as an adjuvant therapy.[40]

ADJUVANT TRIALS OF VASCULAR ENDOTHELIAL GROWTH FACTOR–TARGETED AGENTS

Identification of the genetic basis for RCC in von Hippel-Lindau (VHL) disease led to the discovery that this pathway was also important in sporadic forms of clear cell RCC.[41,42] *VHL* acts as a classic tumor suppressor gene. VHL dysregulation leads to hypoxia inducible factor-α/β accumulation and the transcription of products relating to angiogenesis, glucose transport, and cell cycle regulation.[43,44] A suite of drugs approved for metastatic RCC block the action of the VEGF tyrosine kinases (eg, sorafenib, sunitinib, pazopanib, axitinib, and cabozantinib).[45] Another overlapping pathway resulting in angiogenesis from hypoxic stress involves mammalian target of rapamycin (mTOR), with 2 FDA-approved drugs for RCC (ie, temsirolimus, everolimus).[46–48]

Based on the positive impact of these therapies in metastatic disease, and the high risk and poor prognosis of recurrent/metastatic RCC, a series of randomized placebo-controlled trials beginning in the mid-2000s sought to evaluate tyrosine kinase inhibitors (TKIs) in the adjuvant setting. However, virtually every trial to date has failed to show an improvement in DFS or OS. A single positive trial, the S-TRAC trial,[4] did show a benefit in DFS, but many investigators believe the potential benefits are insufficient to change the standard of care. These trials are briefly reviewed later, and are summarized in **Table 3**.[3–5,49–52]

ASSURE

The ASSURE trial was the largest trial of adjuvant TKIs for high-risk RCC.[3] The trial compared the use of 1 year of adjuvant sorafenib or sunitinib with placebo (1:1:1) and included individuals with intermediate-high or very-high-risk clear cell or non–clear cell RCC. Given toxicity, a dose reduction became standard for all patients to improve tolerability and adherence.

A total of 647 patients were assigned to sunitinib, 649 to sorafenib, and 647 to placebo. After a median follow-up of 5.8 years, the trial was stopped after sufficient events were reached. The primary outcome of the trial, DFS, was not significantly different between groups, including a subanalysis by histology. Similarly, OS did not significantly differ between groups.[3]

Expected adverse effects were common in the active therapeutic arms, including hypertension, hand-foot syndrome, fatigue, and rash/desquamation. Although the midstudy dose reduction significantly reduced patient discontinuation, grade 3 or worse events were still common after the protocol change.

S-TRAC

S-TRAC was an industry-sponsored trial exploring the effect of adjuvant sunitinib in RCC. In this trial, 615 patients with clear cell RCC were randomized to a year of sunitinib versus placebo after surgical resection.[4] Determination of recurrence was made by both investigator assessment as well as a blinded, independent central radiology review (as opposed to ASSURE, which was only by investigator assessment). In this trial, DFS was significantly improved in the sunitinib arm (6.8 vs 5.6 years; HR, 0.76; 95% confidence interval [CI], 0.59–098), a benefit that stands alone as the only survival benefit seen in any of the adjuvant TKI trials. However, OS was not significantly different between the 2 groups at the time of reporting of 5.4 years median follow-up (deaths in 20.7% vs 20.9% in sunitinib and placebo arms, respectively; HR 1.01). Again, the expected toxicity was common for patients in the sunitinib arm (grade 3 and 4 events in 48.4% and 12.1% for the sunitinib arm vs 15.8% and 3.6% for placebo), as were dose reductions and discontinuations (34.3% and 28.1% vs 2% and 5.6% in the sunitinib and placebo arms, respectively). As a result of the DFS benefit, sunitinib did receive FDA approval for this indication. However, owing to the lack of an OS benefit, and the significant side effect profile, several professional organizations have questioned the merit of sunitinib in this setting, and it seems unlikely to be widely used for this indication.[53,54] In a recent update (at 6.6 and 6.7 years median follow-up), DFS continued to be significantly longer in the sunitinib arm (6.2 vs 4.0 years). However, OS data may need more time to mature because of the limited number of events: 67 (21.7%) and 74 (24.2%) patients in each cohort (HR, 0.92; 95% CI, 0.66–1.28).[55]

EVEREST

The EVEREST trial opened in 2010 and randomized 1545 patients with pT1b or pT2-4 completely resected clear cell or papillary RCC to everolimus or placebo for 1 year.[51] RFS is the primary outcome, with secondary outcomes including OS, toxicity profiles, and quality-of-life measures. Trial accrual has closed and final results are expected October 2021.[51]

PROTECT

PROTECT was an industry-sponsored protocol that randomized 1538 patients with pT2 (high grade) or pT3/pT4, pTxN+ clear cell RCC to 1 year of placebo versus pazopanib after surgery. As with other trials, toxicity was an issue, and the 800-mg starting dose of pazopanib was reduced to 600 mg.[49] A total of 403 patients started in the higher-dose randomization (assigned $pazopanib_{800}$ n = 198 vs placebo n = 205) and 1135 at the lower dose ($pazopanib_{600}$ n = 571 vs placebo n = 564).

The primary end point was not met for the ITT_{600} group (HR, 0.86; 95% CI, 0.70–1.06). However, in both the ITT_{800} and ITT_{all} groups, there was a

Table 3
Phase III adjuvant trials using vascular endothelial growth factor/mammalian target of rapamycin pathway targeting agents

	ASSURE	PROTECT	ARISER	ATLAS	S-TRAC	EVEREST	SORCE
Studies	Haas et al,[3] 2016	Motzer et al,[49] 2017	Chamie et al,[5] 2017	Gross-Goupil et al,[50] 2018	Ravaud et al,[4] 2016	S0931[51]	Elsen et al,[52] 2019
Enrollment Dates	April 2006 to Sept 2010	Dec 2010 to Sept 2013	June 2004 to April 2013	May 2012 to July 2016	Sept 2007 to April 2011	May 2010 to Sept 2016	July 2007 to April 2013
N	1943	1538	864	724	615	1545	1711
Status	Complete	Complete	Complete	Complete	DFS data mature (await OS data)	Active (not recruiting)	Complete
Eligibility Criteria	pT2-pT4 pTxN+ pT1 G3/4	pT3-pT4 pT2 G3/4 pTxN+	pT3-pT4 pTxN+ pT1b-pT2 G3/G4	pT2-pT4 pTxN+	pT3-pT4 pTxN+	pT2-pT4 pTxN+ pT1b G3/G4	Leibovich score 3–11
Risk Group (Risk System)	Intermediate or high (UISS)	Intermediate or high (SSIGN)	High (TNM 2002)	Intermediate or high (UISS)	High (UISS)	Intermediate high or high (not specified)	Intermediate or high (Leibovich)
Histology	Clear cell (79%) Non-clear cell (21%)	Clear cell only	Clear cell only	Clear cell only	Clear cell only	Clear cell Non-clear cell	Clear cell (84%) Non-clear cell (16%)
Control Arm	Placebo	Placebo	Placebo	Placebo	Placebo	Placebo	Placebo
Intervention arms	Sunitinib 50 or 37.5 mg daily, 4 wk on, 2 wk off Or Sorafenib 400 or 200 mg twice daily	Pazopanib 600 mg or 800 mg daily	Girentuximab 50 mg ×1, 20 mg weekly	Axitinib 5 mg twice daily	Sunitinib 50 mg 4 wk on, 2 wk off	Everolimus 10 mg daily	Sorafenib 400 mg twice daily for 3 y Or Sorafenib twice daily for 1 y, then placebo for 2 y

Treatment Duration (mo)	12	12	6	12–36	12	12	12–36
Minimum Allowed Dose	Sunitinib 25 mg daily Sorafenib 400 mg every other day	Pazopanib 400 mg daily	No dose reductions	Axitinib 1 mg twice daily	Sunitinib 37.5 mg daily	—	Sorafenib 400 mg daily
Key Efficacy Findings	DFS: HR 1.02, 97.5% CI 0.85–1.23 for sunitinib DFS: HR 0.97, 97.5% CI 0.80–1.17 for sorafenib	ITT$_{600}$: HR 0.86, 95% CI 0.70–1.06 ITT$_{800}$: HR 0.69, 95% CI 0.51–0.94 ITT$_{all}$: HR 0.80, 95% CI 0.68–0.95	DFS: HR 0.97, 95% CI 0.79–1.18 OS: HR 0.99, 95% CI 0.74–1.32	DFS: HR 0.870, 95% CI 0.660–1.147	DFS: HR 0.76, 95% CI 0.59–0.98	Pending	Median DFS not reached for any arm, HR 1.01, 95% CI 0.83–1.23
Trial Conclusion	No benefit for sunitinib or sorafenib	No benefit for pazopanib	No benefit for girentuximab	No benefit for axitinib	DFS benefit for sunitinib, OS data not mature	Pending	No benefit for sorafenib

Abbreviations: CI, confidence interval; TNM, tumor node metastasis.
Data from Refs.[3–5,49–52]

significant improvement in DFS favoring pazopanib at a median follow-up of 47.9 months (ITT$_{800}$ HR, 0.69; 95% CI, 0.51–0.94; and ITT$_{all}$ HR, 0.80; 95% CI, 0.68–0.95). There was no difference in OS at the end of the evaluation period for either dose. Dose reductions and discontinuations were high in both treatment arms. Adverse events were common (98% experienced at least 1) with diarrhea, hypertension, hair color changes, and nausea as the most frequent.

ATLAS

The ATLAS trial was an industry-sponsored trial that randomized patients with predominantly clear cell histology to axitinib 5 mg twice daily or placebo for no less than 1 year and no greater than 3 years.[50] A total of 724 patients in Asia and India were randomized, with independent review committee–assessed DFS as the primary end point. At a preplanned interim analysis after 203 DFS events, the trial was stopped because of futility. Although the trial was negative, a preplanned subgroup analysis of patients at highest risk of recurrence showed a reduction in the risk of DFS events per independent review with an HR 0.735 (95% CI, 0.525–1.028). Dose reductions were required in 56% of the patients receiving axitinib, and more grade 3 and 4 adverse events (61% vs 30%) and discontinuations caused by adverse events (23% vs 11%) were reported for axitinib.

SORCE

The SORCE trial was an industry-sponsored trial enrolling patients with either clear cell or non–clear cell histology and intermediate and high risk of recurrence based on the Leibovich score.[52] Patients were randomized (1:1:1) to placebo, 1 year of sorafenib (followed by 2 years placebo), or 3 years of sorafenib. The investigators observed no differences in DFS or OS in any of the preplanned and prepowered analyses, including all randomized patients, high-risk patients only, and patients with clear cell RCC only. Consistent with other trials, there were high rates of discontinuation because of adverse events from sorafenib, including 24% of patients with grade 3 hand-foot syndrome.

ARISER

An additional adjuvant trial evaluated a monoclonal antibody, girentuximab, which binds to carbonic anhydrase IX (CAIX). CAIX is a cell surface antigen that is highly expressed in most clear cell kidney cancers as a result of dysregulation of VHL.[56] Targeting this protein with monoclonal antibodies showed promise in slowing disease progression in phase I/II trials and was thus identified as a potential agent for use in the adjuvant setting.[57] The ARISER trial was a randomized, double-blind, placebo-controlled trial that evaluated girentuximab as an adjuvant therapy in patients with high-risk clear cell RCC.[5] The trial enrolled 864 patients randomized to placebo versus girentuximab for 6 months. The trial found no benefit to girentuximab treatment in DFS or OS, regardless of pathologic group. Adverse events were rare and not significantly different between the treatment and placebo arms. Despite its promise in earlier trials, the negative results of the ARISER trial have, for now, ended further inquiry into CAIX as a viable target for management of high-risk RCC.

SUMMARIZING THE EVIDENCE FOR ADJUVANT TREATMENT WITH TYROSINE KINASE INHIBITORS/MAMMALIAN TARGET OF RAPAMYCIN INHIBITORS

The results of the adjuvant TKI trials have been widely analyzed, with particular focus on the possible explanations for why the S-TRAC trial found a DFS benefit, whereas the remaining trials, some of which were larger, did not. Various hypotheses have been proposed to explain the divergent results. One explanation is the heterogeneity of inclusion criteria across the studies. S-TRAC had the most restrictive inclusion criteria for the highest-risk individuals, requiring tumors to be at least pT3, whereas ASSURE and both PROTECT and ATLAS all allowed patients with pT1b high-grade and pT2 tumors, respectively. These lower-risk patients comprised approximately one-third of the patient cohort in the ASSURE trial. The assumption is that the presence of these lower-risk patients may have washed out the treatment effect in the higher-risk patients. This potential explanation was evaluated in a post-hoc subset analysis in the ASSURE trial, in which only a high-risk subset of the ASSURE trial that mirrored those patients in the S-TRAC trial (patients with pT3 or pT4 or N+ disease) were analyzed.[7] Despite limiting to this high-risk subset (which was larger than the S-TRAC cohort), they still failed to find a DFS benefit for sunitinib. ATLAS similarly performed a subset analysis on the highest-risk cohort and did show an improvement in DFS.[50] Another potential explanation attributable to differences in inclusion criteria relates to the decision to include non–clear cell histology in the ASSURE trial (representing 20% of the treatment arm), which may be less susceptible to treatment with a TKI.

Table 4
Adjuvant trials using checkpoint inhibitors

	IMMotion 010	Keynote-564	Checkmate 914[67]	Prosper	Rampart[69]
Study	Uzzo et al,[65] 2017	Choueiri et al,[66] 2018	—	Harshman et al,[68] 2019	—
clinicaltrials.gov Identifier	NCT03024996	NCT03142334	NCT03138512	NCT03055013	NCT03288532
Phase	III	III	III	III	III
Status	Active, not recruiting	Active, not recruiting	Recruiting	Recruiting	Recruiting
Sponsor	Hoffmann-La Roche	Merck	Bristol-Myers Squibb	National Cancer Institute	University College, London
Eligibility Criteria	pT2 G4 pT3a G3-4 pT3b/c/T4 pTxN+ M1[a]	pT2 G4 pT3 pT4 pTxN+ M1[a]	pT2a G3/G4 pT2-pT4 pTxN+	cT2-pT4 cTxN+ M1[a]	Leibovich score 3–11
Estimated Enrollment	778	950	800	805	1750
Estimated Completion Date	April 13, 2024	December 28, 2025	July 7, 2023	November 30, 2023	December 1, 2037
Histology	Clear cell or sarcomatoid	Clear cell[b]	Clear cell[b]	Any	Any[c]
Control Arm	Placebo	Placebo	Placebo	Observation	Observation
Intervention arms	Atezolizumab 1200 mg IV q3 wk	Pembrolizumab 200 mg IV q3 wk	Nivolumab + ipilimumab	Nivolumab: 2 doses neoadjuvant Nivo 240 mg, adjuvant Nivo for 9 mo	Durvalumab 1500 mg q4 wk Or Durvalumab 1500 mg q4 wk + tremelimumab

(continued on next page)

Table 4
(continued)

	IMMotion 010	Keynote-564	Checkmate 914[67]	Prosper	Rampart[69]
Treatment Duration (mo)	12	12	6	9	12
Key Efficacy End Points	DFS, OS	DFS, OS	DFS, OS	RFS, OS, OS (cc)	DFS, OS

Abbreviations: IV, intravenous; M1, patients with isolated lung, soft tissue, or nodal metastases that have been completely resected or ablated; OS (cc), OS among patients with clear cell; q, every.

[a] M1 disease allowed if oligometastatic, sites can be definitively treated, and patient rendered NED.

[b] Sarcomatoid features allowed.

[c] Oncocytoma, medullary, collecting duct excluded.

Data from Refs.[65–69]

Rampart column header: 75 mg on day 1 and week 4

Another possible explanation for result differences were differences in drug exposure between the trials. In all of the trials of TKI, dose reductions were allowed, but the minimum allowed dosages differed between trials. Data from advanced kidney cancer studies with TKIs such as axitinib show that there is variability in drug exposure and higher levels may be associated with improved response.[58] In S-TRAC, many patients remained on sunitinib at 50 mg/d, whereas, in ASSURE, poor tolerability led to the protocol being amended to 37.5 mg/d. Although ASSURE could have been hampered by inadequate drug exposure,[3,59] an additional subset analysis of patients having the highest quartile of sunitinib dose did not show any improvement in outcome. Data from the PROTECT trial also suggest that higher drug exposure leads to better drug efficacy; however, similar to ASSURE, there was dose reduction early on because of tolerability (from 800 to 600 mg of pazopanib).[7]

Based on the S-TRAC data, adjuvant sunitinib was brought for regulatory approval in the United States. The FDA Oncologic Drug Advisory Committee had a split vote (6 to 6) but the agent was approved.[60] Neither The Kidney Cancer Research Network of Canada nor the European Association of Urology support routine use of TKIs in the adjuvant setting,[53,54] and the current NCCN guidelines continue to support enrollment in clinical trials as the preferred management strategy for patients with stage 2 and 3 disease. Given the heterogeneity of findings of the adjuvant TKI trials, as well as the toxicity, there is a general consensus that, although adjuvant sunitinib should be discussed, it is not the standard of care for all patients following nephrectomy.

CHECKPOINT INHIBITION IN THE LOCALIZED DISEASE STATE

Inhibition of immune checkpoint tolerance pathways has been shown to produce durable responses and improve survival in several malignancies in the advanced disease state, including RCC. In kidney cancer, nivolumab was first approved after OS benefit was seen compared with everolimus in the second-line setting.[61] Since then, inhibition of the programmed cell death protein 1 (PD-1)/programmed death-ligand 1 (PD-L1) pathway has become a central component in the treatment of advanced disease, both as monotherapy in the second-line setting and in combination with cytotoxic T lymphocyte–associated protein 4 (CTLA-4) inhibition (ipilimumab) or with TKI (axitinib) in the first-line setting.[62,63]

Checkpoint inhibition has been shown to augment the immune response, resulting in cytotoxicity to tumor cells. This direct cytotoxicity may ultimately be more effective at eliminating residual microscopic cancer cells compared with VEGF inhibition, which relies on inhibiting angiogenesis, which may not be a critical part of the biology of micrometastases. Checkpoint inhibition is a proven viable adjuvant treatment in other malignancies, such as melanoma, where it has been shown to improve RFS in completely resected melanoma at high risk for recurrence.[64] In RCC, there are several ongoing clinical trials with checkpoint inhibitors used in the adjuvant setting. These trials differ slightly in inclusion criteria, histology, timing of therapy, as well as the specific agents (Table 4).[65–69] A classic adjuvant therapy design is used in several trials using PD-1/PD-L1 therapy within the first 8 to 12 weeks after surgery for predominantly clear cell or sarcomatoid-transformed RCC. Agents in these trials include pembrolizumab (NCT03142334), durvalumab (NCT03288532), atezolizumab (NCT03024996), and combination therapy with ipilimumab and nivolumab (NCT03138512). The ipilimumab and nivolumab trial is currently undergoing an amendment to allow a monotherapy nivolumab arm.

Training the immune system to recognize residual cells may require the presence of a significant volume of antigen. Treatment in the neoadjuvant (vs adjuvant) phase may allow greater stimulation and promotion of effective tumor-infiltrating lymphocytes and improved immune response because the primary tumor, and its antigenic targets, remain in place at that time. The PROSPER RCC trial (NCT03055013) is a cooperative group trial evaluating a single dose of nivolumab before surgery followed by classic adjuvant therapy for up to a year.[68] This trial differs from pure adjuvant trials because there is no placebo control, and the single dose given in the neoadjuvant phase allows for initial immune priming.

SUMMARY

For patients who undergo surgery for high-risk, clinically localized kidney cancer, approximately half recur in the 6 years following surgery. Adjuvant therapy has been shown to be an effective treatment strategy in a host of solid tumor types, and has been extensively investigated in kidney cancer. However, despite a large number of trials evaluating agents with known biological activity against kidney cancer, only a single trial has shown a DFS benefit when used as an adjuvant therapy to surgery, and has yet to show a benefit in OS. Although sunitinib is FDA approved for this indication, given the questionable benefit and substantial toxicity, it is unlikely to be widely used. A variety of monoclonal antibodies targeting checkpoint inhibition pathways are now being investigated in the adjuvant and combination neo/adjuvant setting, and initial results are expected in the next 3 to 5 years. Until an effective adjuvant therapy is developed, risk-adapted observation remains the standard following surgery, and enrollment of patients at high risk for recurrence in clinical trials is strongly encouraged.

DISCLOSURE

The authors have nothing to disclose.

REFERENCES

1. Patel HD, Gupta M, Joice GA, et al. Clinical stage migration and survival for renal cell carcinoma in the United States. Eur Urol Oncol 2019;2(4):343–8.
2. Syed JS, Nawaf CF, Rosoff J, et al. Adverse pathologic characteristics in the small renal mass: implications for active surveillance. - Abstract - Europe PMC. Available at: https://europepmc.org/article/med/28436365. Accessed January 6, 2020.
3. Haas NB, Manola J, Uzzo RG, et al. Adjuvant sunitinib or sorafenib for high-risk, non-metastatic renal-cell carcinoma (ECOG-ACRIN E2805): a double-blind, placebo-controlled, randomised, phase 3 trial. Lancet 2016;387(10032):2008–16.
4. Ravaud A, Motzer RJ, Pandha HS, et al. Adjuvant sunitinib in high-risk renal-cell carcinoma after nephrectomy. N Engl J Med 2016;375(23):2246–54.
5. Chamie K, Donin NM, Klöpfer P, et al. Adjuvant weekly girentuximab following nephrectomy for high-risk renal cell carcinoma: the ARISER randomized clinical trial. JAMA Oncol 2017;3(7):913–20.
6. Lam John S, Oleg S, Leppert John T, et al. Postoperative surveillance protocol for patients with localized and locally advanced renal cell carcinoma based on a validated prognostic nomogram and risk group stratification system. J Urol 2005;174(2):466–72.
7. Haas NB, Manola J, Dutcher JP, et al. Adjuvant treatment for high-risk clear cell renal cancer: updated results of a high-risk subset of the ASSURE randomized trial. JAMA Oncol 2017;3(9):1249–52.
8. Motzer RJ, Jonasch E, Agarwal N, et al. NCCN Guidelines: Kidney Cancer. Kidney Cancer, Version 2 2019;64.
9. Wood Erika L, Adibi M, Qiao Wei, et al. Local tumor bed recurrence following partial nephrectomy in patients with small renal masses. J Urol 2018;199(2):393–400.
10. Abara E, Chivulescu I, Clerk N, et al. Recurrent renal cell cancer: 10 years or more after nephrectomy. Can Urol Assoc J 2010;4(2):E45–9.
11. Eggener SE, Yossepowitch O, Pettus JA, et al. Renal cell carcinoma recurrence after nephrectomy for localized disease: predicting survival from time of recurrence. J Clin Oncol 2006;24(19):3101–6.
12. Chin AI, Lam JS, Figlin RA, et al. Surveillance strategies for renal cell carcinoma patients following nephrectomy. Rev Urol 2006;8(1):1–7.
13. Shuch BM, Lam JS, Belldegrun AS, et al. Prognostic factors in renal cell carcinoma. Semin Oncol 2006;33(5):563–75.
14. Nguyen DP, Vertosick EA, Corradi RB, et al. Histological subtype of renal cell carcinoma significantly impacts survival in the era of partial nephrectomy. Urol Oncol 2016;34(6):259.e1-e8.
15. Patard J-J, Leray E, Rioux-Leclercq N, et al. Prognostic Value of Histologic Subtypes in Renal Cell Carcinoma: A Multicenter Experience. J Clin Oncol 2005;23(12):2763–71. https://doi.org/10.1200/JCO.2005.07.055.
16. Leibovich Bradley C, Lohse Christine M, Crispen Paul L, et al. Histological subtype is an independent predictor of outcome for patients with renal cell carcinoma. J Urol 2010;183(4):1309–16.
17. Zisman A, Pantuck AJ, Wieder J, et al. Risk group assessment and clinical outcome algorithm to predict the natural history of patients with surgically resected renal cell carcinoma. J Clin Oncol 2002;20(23):4559–66.
18. Frank I, Blute ML, Cheville JC, et al. An outcome prediction model for patients with clear cell renal cell carcinoma treated with radical nephrectomy based on tumor stage, size, grade and necrosis: the SSIGN score. J Urol 2002;168(6):2395–400.
19. Leibovich BC, Blute ML, Cheville JC, et al. Prediction of progression after radical nephrectomy for patients with clear cell renal cell carcinoma. Cancer 2003;97(7):1663–71.
20. Kattan MW, Reuter V, Motzer RJ, et al. A postoperative prognostic nomogram for renal cell carcinoma. J Urol 2001;166(1):63–7.
21. Raj GV, Houston TR, Leibovich Bradley C, et al. Preoperative nomogram predicting 12-year probability of metastatic renal cancer. J Urol 2008;179(6):2146–51.
22. Shuch B, Pantuck AJ, Pouliot F, et al. Quality of pathological reporting for renal cell cancer: implications for systemic therapy, prognostication and surveillance. BJU Int 2011;108(3):343–8.
23. Klatte T, Seligson DB, LaRochelle J, et al. Molecular signatures of localized clear cell renal cell carcinoma to predict disease-free survival after nephrectomy. Cancer Epidemiol Biomarkers Prev 2009;18(3):894–900.
24. Hanahan D, Folkman J. Patterns and emerging mechanisms of the angiogenic switch during tumorigenesis. Cell 1996;86(3):353–64.

25. Chism DD, Rathmell WK. Kidney cancer: Rest ASSUREd, much can be learned from adjuvant studies in renal cancer. Nat Rev Nephrol 2016; 12(6):317–8.

26. Suciu S, Eggermont AMM, Lorigan P, et al. Relapse-free survival as a surrogate for overall survival in the evaluation of stage II-III melanoma adjuvant therapy. J Natl Cancer Inst 2018;110(1). https://doi.org/10.1093/jnci/djx133.

27. Sargent DJ, Wieand HS, Haller DG, et al. Disease-free survival versus overall survival as a primary end point for adjuvant colon cancer studies: individual patient data from 20,898 patients on 18 randomized trials. J Clin Oncol 2005;23(34): 8664–70.

28. Hess LM, Brnabic A, Mason O, et al. Relationship between Progression-free Survival and Overall Survival in Randomized Clinical Trials of Targeted and Biologic Agents in Oncology. J Cancer 2019; 10(16):3717–27.

29. Becker A, Eichelberg C, Sun M. Progression-free survival: Does a correlation with survival justify its role as a surrogate clinical endpoint? Cancer 2014; 120(1):7–10.

30. Bukowski RM. Natural history and therapy of metastatic renal cell carcinoma. Cancer 1997;80(7): 1198–220.

31. Pantuck Allan J, Amnon Z, Belldegrun Arie S. The changing natural history of renal cell carcinoma. J Urol 2001;166(5):1611–23.

32. Fyfe G, Fisher RI, Rosenberg SA, et al. Results of treatment of 255 patients with metastatic renal cell carcinoma who received high-dose recombinant interleukin-2 therapy. J Clin Oncol 1995;13(3): 688–96.

33. Allard CB, Gelpi-Hammerschmidt F, Harshman LC, et al. Contemporary trends in high-dose interleukin-2 use for metastatic renal cell carcinoma in the United States. Urol Oncol 2015;33(11). 496. e11-e16.

34. Klapper JA, Downey SG, Smith FO, et al. High-dose interleukin-2 for the treatment of metastatic renal cell carcinoma. Cancer 2008;113(2):293–301.

35. Pizzocaro G, Piva L, Colavita M, et al. Interferon adjuvant to radical nephrectomy in robson stages II and III renal cell carcinoma: a multicentric randomized study. J Clin Oncol 2001;19(2):425–31.

36. Messing EM, Manola J, Wilding G, et al. Phase III Study of Interferon Alfa-NL as adjuvant treatment for resectable renal cell carcinoma: an eastern cooperative oncology group/intergroup trial. J Clin Oncol 2003;21(7):1214–22.

37. Clark JI, Atkins MB, Urba WJ, et al. Adjuvant High-Dose Bolus Interleukin-2 for Patients With High-Risk Renal Cell Carcinoma: A Cytokine Working Group Randomized Trial. J Clin Oncol 2003;21(16): 3133–40.

38. Jocham D, Richter A, Hoffmann L, et al. Adjuvant autologous renal tumour cell vaccine and risk of tumour progression in patients with renal-cell carcinoma after radical nephrectomy: phase III, randomised controlled trial. Lancet 2004;363(9409): 594–9.

39. Wood C, Srivastava P, Bukowski R, et al. An adjuvant autologous therapeutic vaccine (HSPPC-96; vitespen) versus observation alone for patients at high risk of recurrence after nephrectomy for renal cell carcinoma: a multicentre, open-label, randomised phase III trial. Lancet 2008;372(9633): 145–54.

40. Milestone: Kidney Cancer Vaccine Oncophage Approved in Russia. Cancer Research Institute. Available at: https://www.cancerresearch.org/news/2008/milestone-kidney-cancer-vaccine-oncophage-approved. Accessed January 27, 2020.

41. Latif F, Tory K, Gnarra J, et al. Identification of the von Hippel-Lindau disease tumor suppressor gene. Science 1993;260(5112):1317–20.

42. Gnarra JR, Tory K, Weng Y, et al. Mutations of the VHL tumour suppressor gene in renal carcinoma. Nat Genet 1994;7(1):85–90.

43. Ma X, Yang K, Lindblad P, et al. VHL gene alterations in renal cell carcinoma patients: novel hotspot or founder mutations and linkage disequilibrium. Oncogene 2001;20(38):5393–400.

44. Creighton CJ, Morgan M, Gunaratne PH, et al. Comprehensive molecular characterization of clear cell renal cell carcinoma. Nature 2013;499(7456): 43–9.

45. Vachhani P, George S. VEGF inhibitors in renal cell carcinoma. Clin Adv Hematol Oncol 2016;14(12): 1016–28.

46. Kapoor A, Figlin RA. Targeted inhibition of mammalian target of rapamycin for the treatment of advanced renal cell carcinoma. Cancer 2009; 115(16):3618–30.

47. Guertin DA, Sabatini DM. The Pharmacology of mTOR Inhibition. Sci Signal 2009;2(67):pe24.

48. Hudes G, Carducci M, Tomczak P, et al. Temsirolimus, Interferon Alfa, or Both for Advanced Renal-Cell Carcinoma. N Engl J Med 2007;356(22): 2271–81. Available at: https://www.nejm.org/doi/full/10.1056/NEJMoa066838. Accessed December 16, 2019.

49. Motzer RJ, Haas NB, Donskov F, et al. Randomized phase III trial of adjuvant pazopanib versus placebo after nephrectomy in patients with localized or locally advanced renal cell carcinoma. J Clin Oncol 2017. https://doi.org/10.1200/JCO.2017.73.5324.

50. Gross-Goupil M, Kwon TG, Eto M, et al. Axitinib versus placebo as an adjuvant treatment of renal cell carcinoma: results from the phase III, randomized ATLAS trial. Ann Oncol 2018;29(12): 2371–8.

51. S0931, Everolimus in Treating Patients With Kidney Cancer Who Have Undergone Surgery - Full Text View - ClinicalTrials.gov. Available at: https://clinicaltrials.gov/ct2/show/NCT01120249. Accessed January 13, 2020.

52. Eisen TQG, Frangou E, Smith B, et al. LBA56Primary efficacy analysis results from the SORCE trial (RE05): Adjuvant sorafenib for renal cell carcinoma at intermediate or high risk of relapse: An international, randomised double-blind phase III trial led by the MRC CTU at UCL. Ann Oncol 2019; 30(Supplement_5). https://doi.org/10.1093/annonc/mdz394.050.

53. Ljungberg B, Albiges L, Abu-Ghanem Y, et al. European association of urology guidelines on renal cell carcinoma: the 2019 update. Eur Urol 2019;75(5): 799–810.

54. Karakiewicz PI, Zaffuto E, Kapoor A, et al. Kidney Cancer Research Network of Canada consensus statement on the role of adjuvant therapy after nephrectomy for high-risk, non-metastatic renal cell carcinoma: A comprehensive analysis of the literature and meta-analysis of randomized controlled trials. Can Urol Assoc J 2018;12(6):173–80.

55. Motzer RJ, Ravaud A, Patard J-J, et al. Adjuvant sunitinib for high-risk renal cell carcinoma after nephrectomy: subgroup analyses and updated overall survival results. Eur Urol 2018;73(1):62–8.

56. Bui MHT, Seligson D, Han K, et al. Carbonic anhydrase IX is an independent predictor of survival in advanced renal clear cell carcinoma: implications for prognosis and therapy. Clin Cancer Res 2003; 9(2):802–11.

57. Siebels M, Rohrmann K, Oberneder R, et al. A clinical phase I/II trial with the monoclonal antibody cG250 (RENCAREX®) and interferon-alpha-2a in metastatic renal cell carcinoma patients. World J Urol 2011;29(1):121–6.

58. Schmidinger M, Danesi R, Jones R, et al. Individualized dosing with axitinib: rationale and practical guidance. Future Oncol 2017;14(9):861–75.

59. Houk BE, Bello CL, Poland B, et al. Relationship between exposure to sunitinib and efficacy and tolerability endpoints in patients with cancer: results of a pharmacokinetic/pharmacodynamic meta-analysis. Cancer Chemother Pharmacol 2010;66(2): 357–71.

60. September 19, 2017. FDA advisory committee split on opinion of adjuvant Sutent for renal cell carcinoma. Available at: https://www.healio.com/hematology-oncology/genitourinary-cancer/news/online/{664873e9-5a21-43af-bfbe-934cd8417e3f}/fda-advisory-committee-split-on-opinion-of-adjuvant-sutent-for-renal-cell-carcinoma. Accessed April 10, 2020.

61. Motzer RJ, Escudier B, McDermott DF, et al. Nivolumab versus Everolimus in Advanced Renal-Cell Carcinoma. N Engl J Med 2015;373(19):1803–13.

62. Motzer RJ, Rini BI, McDermott DF, et al. Nivolumab plus ipilimumab versus sunitinib in first-line treatment for advanced renal cell carcinoma: extended follow-up of efficacy and safety results from a randomised, controlled; phase 3 trial. Lancet Oncol 2019;20(10):1370–85.

63. Motzer RJ, Penkov K, Haanen J, et al. Avelumab plus Axitinib versus Sunitinib for Advanced Renal-Cell Carcinoma. N Engl J Med 2019;380(12): 1103–15.

64. Eggermont AMM, Blank CU, Mandala M, et al. Adjuvant Pembrolizumab versus Placebo in Resected Stage III Melanoma. N Engl J Med 2018;378(19): 1789–801.

65. Uzzo R, Bex A, Rini BI, et al. A phase III study of atezolizumab (atezo) vs placebo as adjuvant therapy in renal cell carcinoma (RCC) patients (pts) at high risk of recurrence following resection (IMmotion010). J Clin Oncol 2017;35(15_suppl):TPS4598.

66. Choueiri TK, Quinn DI, Zhang T, et al. KEYNOTE-564: A phase 3, randomized, double blind, trial of pembrolizumab in the adjuvant treatment of renal cell carcinoma. J Clin Oncol 2018;36(15_suppl): TPS4599.

67. A Study Comparing the Combination of Nivolumab and Ipilimumab Versus Placebo in Participants With Localized Renal Cell Carcinoma - Full Text View - ClinicalTrials.gov. Available at: https://clinicaltrials.gov/ct2/show/NCT03138512. Accessed February 21, 2020.

68. Harshman LC, Puligandla M, Haas NB, et al. PROSPER: A phase III randomized study comparing perioperative nivolumab (nivo) versus observation in patients with localized renal cell carcinoma (RCC) undergoing nephrectomy (ECOG-ACRIN 8143). J Clin Oncol 2019;37(7_suppl):TPS684.

69. Renal Adjuvant MultiPle Arm Randomised Trial - Full Text View - ClinicalTrials.gov. Available at: https://clinicaltrials.gov/ct2/show/NCT03288532. Accessed February 21, 2020.

Cytoreductive Nephrectomy in the Era of Tyrosine Kinase and Immuno-Oncology Checkpoint Inhibitors

Michael J. Biles, MD*, Hiten D. Patel, MD, MPH, Mohamad E. Allaf, MD

KEYWORDS

• Kidney cancer • Renal cell carcinoma • Cytoreductive nephrectomy • Systemic therapy

KEY POINTS

• The role of cytoreductive nephrectomy (CN) in the management of metastatic renal cell carcinoma (mRCC) continues to evolve with advancements in systemic therapy.
• Although CN previously was standard of care for all patients with mRCC, the vascular endothelial growth factor (VEGF)-targeted therapy era highlighted the importance of systemic therapy in improving oncologic outcomes and the importance of risk stratification to identify patients more likely to benefit from CN.
• Immuno-oncology (IO) checkpoint inhibitors and combination IO and VEGF-targeted therapy agents (IOVE) currently are transforming the management of mRCC.
• CN continues to play an important role in specific patient populations, including those with low-volume, favorable-risk mRCC and those with stable or regressive disease on systemic therapy, and in delaying initiation of toxic systemic therapy in patients who can be observed.
• The role of CN needs to be re-examined in the new IO/IOVE era.

INTRODUCTION

Renal cell carcinoma (RCC) is the twelfth most common cancer. In the United States, in 2019, there were approximately 74,000 new cases diagnosed and 15,000 deaths.[1] The incidence has increased with routine use of imaging modalities, increasing the number of incidentally diagnosed renal malignancies, which has resulted in stage migration, leading to approximately 70% of newly detected kidney tumors being low stage, clinically localized (cT1) renal masses.[2] Historically, 25% to 30% of patients presented with distant metastases, but with earlier detection the current metastatic rate at presentation is closer to 10% to 15% in the United States and Europe.[3–7] Disseminated disease still carries a dismal prognosis, with 5-year survival rates at approximately 10%, although survival rates over the past 30 years have improved with the advent of novel targeted therapies.[3,8–11]

Extirpative surgery has been a primary treatment option for patients with locally advanced, lymph node–positive, and distant metastatic RCC (mRCC), although its role in metastatic disease continues to evolve with advancements in

Financial Disclosures/Funding Source: None.
James Buchanan Brady Urological Institute, The Johns Hopkins Medical Institutions, 600 N. Wolfe Street / Marburg 144, Baltimore, MD 21287, USA
* Corresponding author.
E-mail address: mbiles1@jhmi.edu

Urol Clin N Am 47 (2020) 359–370
https://doi.org/10.1016/j.ucl.2020.04.009

urologic.theclinics.com

systemic therapy.[12,13] Cytoreductive nephrectomy (CN) refers to the removal of the kidney with the primary tumor in patients with synchronous mRCC. During the cytokine therapy era, CN provided a clear survival benefit in patients with metastatic disease.[14–16] The development of targeted therapies, such as tyrosine kinase inhibitors (TKIs), vascular endothelial growth factor (VEGF) monoclonal antibodies, and mammalian target of rapamycin (mTOR) inhibitors, have made the indications for CN less clear, and the recent advent of novel immune-oncologic (IO) agents have blurred its value further.

New efforts have been made to define the indications for CN, considering patient characteristics and disease pathology, the oncologic benefits of surgical management compared with modern systemic therapy, and the morbidity of surgery. Exploration into the timing of CN in relation to systemic therapy also is needed. This article aims to critically review the current literature to provide guidance on the therapeutic role of CN, including patient selection and surgical timing, in treating patients with mRCC in the modern systemic therapy era.

BENEFIT OF CYTOREDUCTIVE THERAPY ALONE IN METASTATIC RENAL CELL CARCINOMA

CN until recently has been considered standard of care for all patients with mRCC. Its mechanism in altering the course of disease is unclear, but the pathophysiologic benefit likely is multifactorial. The elimination of the primary tumor reduces disease burden and the potential for development of aggressive biological clones capable of metastases.[17] RCC is known to be highly immunogenic, and CN has been proposed to alter the immune systems response to metastases. In the early 1990s, prior to Food and Drug Administration approval of interleukin (IL)-2, CN alone was observed to result in spontaneous regression of distant metastatic lesions in a minority of patients.[18–20] Although cure in these cases is rare and unpredictable even with risk stratification, the witnessed abscopal effect led to the realization of RCC immunogenicity. In theory, the immune system may be primed to target renal cancer cells, but the response is consumed by the primary tumor until it is removed, possibly due to the volume of disease or the immunosuppressive nature of the tumor microenvironment, inhibiting T-cell function.[21,22] Recent clinical studies have demonstrated correlation of RCC metastatic immunogenicity, in particular pulmonary and skeletal metastases, with clinical outcome.[23,24] CN had a theoretic basis to

improve survival in patients with mRCC, by removing a potential source for new metastases and freeing the immune system to combat existing metastatic disease.[25]

CYTOKINE-BASED IMMUNOTHERAPY ERA

The recognition of RCC's immunogenicity led to the evaluation of immunotherapy, including IL-2 and interferon (IFN)-α, in treating metastatic disease.[26] In 2001, the Southwest Oncology Group (SWOG) and European Organisation for Research and Treatment of Cancer (EORTC) published 2 randomized controlled trials (RCTs) with nearly identical protocols, randomizing patients with mRCC to CN followed by IFN-α or to IFN-α alone (**Table 1**).[14,15] Both studies demonstrated improved overall survival in patients receiving surgery plus immunotherapy. SWOG 8949 included 241 total patients and showed an improved median overall survival of 3 months (11.1 mo vs 8.1 mo respectively; P = .05).[14] EORTC 30947 included 85 total patients and had a difference in median overall survival of 10 months (17 mo vs 7 mo respectively; P = .03).[15] A combined analyses of these 2 trials with 331 patients showed an improved median survival of 13.6 months in the CN plus IFN-α group in comparison to 7.8 months for IFN-α alone (31% decrease in the risk of death), independent of performance status and metastatic site.[16] When evaluating CN in mRCC, it is important to note the percentage of patients who actually receive systemic therapy, because surgery can consequently delay initiation of or eliminate the possibility of systemic treatment. In these trials, only 1.8% of patients in the IFN-α–only arm did not receive IFN-α, whereas 5.6% of patients in the combined treatment arm did not receive IFN-α after nephrectomy. Therefore, CN improved overall survival despite fewer patients receiving systemic treatment. This combined analysis led to the conclusion that CN significantly improves overall survival in patients receiving IFN-α.[16]

After these trials, CN with cytokine therapy became standard of care in surgical candidates with synchronous mRCC. Despite the limited survival advantage, however, overall outcomes remained poor, emphasizing the need for more effective systemic treatments.

RISK STRATIFICATION AND PATIENT SELECTION

Metastatic RCC is a disease spectrum encompassing varied pathology at presentation and diverse natural history. As SWOG 8949 and

Table 1
Summary of randomized control studies in metastatic renal cell carcinoma

Trial Name	Authors	N	Memorial Sloan Kettering Cancer Center or International Metastatic Renal Cell Carcinoma Database Consortium Risk Category					Arms		Outcomes		Notes
			Favorable	Inter-mediate	Poor	Un-known	Arm	Arm Description	Complete Response, Partial Response, or Objective Response Rate	Survival (Median Survival, Overall Survival, Progression-Free Survival)	
SWOG 8949	Flanigan et al,[14] 2001	241	—	—	—	241	Arm 1	CN followed by IFN-α	—	MS 11.1 mo	
							Arm 2	IFN-α	—	MS 8.1 mo	
EORTC 30947	Mickisch et al,[15] 2001	85	—	—	—	85	Arm 1	CN followed by IFN-α	CR 11.9%	MS 17 mo	
							Arm 2	IFN-α	CR 2.3%	MS 7 mo	
N/A	Motzer et al[8]	750	264	421	48	0	Arm 1	Sunitinib	OR 31%	Median PFS 11 mo	MSKCC
							Arm 2	IFN-α	OR 6%	Median PFS 5 mo	
Global ARCC Trial	Hudes et al,[36] 2007	626	0	164	462	0	Arm 1	Temsirolimus	OR 8.6%	MS 10.9 mo	
							Arm 2	IFN-α	OR 4.8%	MS 7.3 mo	

(continued on next page)

Table 1
(continued)

Trial Name	Authors	N	Memorial Sloan Kettering Cancer Center or International Metastatic Renal Cell Carcinoma Database Consortium Risk Category				Arms		Outcomes		Notes
			Favorable	Inter-mediate	Poor	Un-known	Arm	Arm Description	Complete Response, Partial Response, or Objective Response Rate	Survival (Median Survival, Overall Survival, Progression-Free Survival)	
TARGET Study	Escudier et al,[12] 2016	903	461	441	0	1	Arm 1	Sorafenib	PR 10%	MS 17.8 mo, PFS 5.5 mo	MSKCC; 48% of patients in placebo group crossed over to receive sorafenib
							Arm 2	Placebo	PR 2%	MS 14.3 mo, PFS 2.8 mo	
CARMENA	Mejean et al,[52] 2018	450	0	256	193	0	Arm 1	CN + sunitinib	OR 27.4%; CR 0.6%	MS 13.9 mo	MSKCC
							Arm 2	Sunitinib	OR 29.1%; CR 0%	MS 18.4 mo	
SURTIME	De Bruijn et al,[56] 2019	99	0	87	12	0	Arm 1	Sunitinib + deferred CN	—	MS 32.4 mo	MSKCC
							Arm 2	Immediate CN + Sunitinib	—	MS 15.1 mo	

Check-Mate 214	Motzer et al[59]	1096	249	847 (intermediate risk or poor risk)	0	Arm 1	Ipi-nivo	OR 42%; CR 11%	MS not reached	IMDC	CheckMate 214
						Arm 2	Sunitinib	OR 29%; CR 2%	MS 26.6 mo		
KEY-NOTE-426	Rini et al[64]	861	269	484	108	0	Arm 1	Pembrolizumab + axitinib	OR 59.3%; CR 5.8%	-y OS 89.9%; PFS 15.1 mo	IMDC
							Arm 2	Sunitinib	OR 35.7%; CR 1.9%	1-y OS 78.3%; PFS 11.1 mo	IMDC

Abbreviations: CR, complete response; MS, median survival; OR, objective response; OS, overall survival; PFS, progression-free survival; PR, partial response.
Data from Refs.[14,15,55,58,59,61–63]

EORTC 30947 demonstrate, trials with similar entry criteria may result in disparate outcomes, possibly attributable to dissimilar sample sizes or significant differences in baseline disease severity despite randomization. Risk stratification is vital to counsel patients and choose treatments that align with patient goals. Several models have been developed based on functional status and serum factors to prognosticate outcomes, guide treatment strategies, and evaluate therapeutic plans.

The Memorial Sloan Kettering Cancer Center (MSKCC) model, also known as the Motzer criteria, was published in 1999 during the immunotherapy era (Table 2).[11] It stratifies patients into 3 risk classifications, including favorable risk, intermediate risk, and poor risk, based on time to initiation of systemic therapy, Karnofsky performance scale status, and serum hemoglobin, calcium, and lactate dehydrogenase levels. During the targeted therapy era, the International Metastatic Renal Cell Carcinoma Database Consortium (IMDC), or Heng criteria, was created, separating patients into the same 3 categories based on prognostic factors for overall survival in patients with mRCC treated with VEGF-TKI. IMDC is similar to MSKCC criteria except for the elimination of serum lactic acid dehydrogenase and the inclusion of neutrophil and platelet counts.[27] The performance of the IMDC model was found similar to that of the MSKCC criteria (see Table 2).[28]

Other studies have identified important risk stratification factors that can be categorized broadly into patient and tumor characteristics. These include metastatic site and burden, cardiopulmonary function, performance status, sarcomatoid features, lymph node involvement, hypoalbuminemia, sarcopenia, and neutrophil-to-lymphocyte ratio.[29–35] The importance of these risk factors is less understood. The MSKCC and IMDC models remain the 2 most widely adopted and validated risk stratification criteria utilized in clinical trials.

VASCULAR ENDOTHELIAL GROWTH FACTOR–TARGETED THERAPY ERA

VEGF-targeted therapies improved outcomes and changed the treatment paradigm for mRCC. VEGF-TKIs, such as sunitinib and sorafenib, and mTOR kinases, such as temsirolimus, were introduced in the early 2000s with superior efficacy in comparison to previous systemic therapy. Sunitinib was approved by the Food and Drug Administration in 2006 and quickly became the new standard of care for mRCC.

Three RCTs were published in 2007, evaluating the new VEGF-targeted agents in patients with mRCC (see **Table 1**). In these trials, patients randomized to receive sunitinib or temsirolimus demonstrated improved overall survival in direct comparison to patients randomized to IFN-α (sunitinib, 11 mo, vs IFN, 5 mo, and temsirolimus, 10.9, mo vs IFN, 7.3 mo).[7,36] In a separate trial, sorafenib was shown to prolong progression-free survival in comparison to placebo (5.5 mo vs 2.8 mo, respectively) in patients who had failed previous systemic therapy.[37] These trials altered the landscape of systemic treatment, highlighting the improved efficacy of targeted therapy over IFN-α immunotherapy. A majority of patients enrolled in these trials had undergone prior nephrectomy, typically with curative intent prior to the development of metachronous metastases.[38] There are few cases of sustained complete responses with targeted therapy in patients with mRCC without primary nephrectomy or CN.[39] As systemic therapy with targeted agents increased, the utilization of CN decreased, because its importance in conjunction with improved systemic therapy was unclear.[40]

Retrospective studies attempted to determine if CN provided an independent survival benefit to patients in the VEGF-TKI era. These studies unanimously showed overall survival benefit in patients receiving CN with targeted therapy in comparison to targeted therapy alone.[41–49] Choueiri and colleagues[41] found a median overall survival of 19.8 months in the CN combination treatment group versus 9.4 months (unadjusted hazard ratio [HR] 0.44 [95% CI, 0.32–0.59]; $P < .01$) in the VEGF-targeted therapy–only group. A large population study evaluating data from the Surveillance, Epidemiology, and End Results (SEER) database, including more than 20,000 patients, found a survival advantage of 19 months versus 4 months respectively in patients receiving combination CN with VEGF-targeted therapy versus targeted therapy alone.[42] A more recent meta-analysis of 11 nonrandomized trials evaluating approximately 40,000 patients with advanced RCC found a 54% reduced risk of death in combination therapy versus targeted therapy alone.[50] Interpreting the data from these retrospective studies is difficult and fraught with inherent biases. Statistically significant differences in baseline group characteristics tended to favor the CN patient populations, including younger age, better performance status, fewer metastases, and improved MSKCC and IMDC risk criteria.[51] This is not surprising because patients selected for surgery tend to be healthier and with more favorable disease. When patients were stratified by risk on subgroup analyses, favorable-risk and intermediate-risk patients tended to drive surgical benefit, whereas patients

Table 2
Memorial Sloan Kettering Cancer Center and International Metastatic Renal Cell Carcinoma Database Consortium risk criteria

Criteria	Memorial Sloan Kettering Cancer Center	International Metastatic Renal Cell Carcinoma Database Consortium
Time from diagnosis to systemic treatment	If <1 y: 1 point	If <1 y: 1 point
Karnofsky performance scale status	If <80%: 1 point	If <80%: 1 point
Hemoglobin	If < lower limit of normal: 1 point Men (normal): 13.5–17.5 g/dL Women (normal): 12.0–15.5 g/dL	If <lower limit of normal: 1 point Normal: usually ~12 g/dL
Calcium	If >10 mg/dL (>2.5 mmol/L): 1 point	If corrected Ca > upper limit of normal: 1 point Normal: ~8.5–10.2 mg/dL
Lactic acid dehydrogenase	If >1.5× upper limit of normal: 1 point Normal: 140 U/L	N/A
Neutrophils	N/A	If > upper limit of normal: 1 point Normal: ~ $2.0 \times$–7.0×10^9/L
Platelets	N/A	If > upper limit of normal: 1 point Normal: 150,000–400,000 cells/μL
Favorable risk	0 points	0 points
Intermediate risk	1–2 points	1–2 points
High/poor risk	3–5 points	3–6 points

Data from Refs.[11,28]

with poor risk seemed to have less or no benefit from CN.[41,47] Prior to the reporting of level 1 evidence, these studies helped provide guidance on patient populations that were more likely to have benefit from CN.

Cancer du Rein Métastatique Nephrectomie et Antiangiogéniques (CARMENA) was a pivotal study published in 2018 conducted to determine more definitively the role of CN in the targeted therapy era (see **Table 1**). It was a phase III, randomized controlled noninferiority trial that included 450 patients with MSKCC intermediate-risk or poor-risk clear cell mRCC randomized to undergo CN followed by sunitinib versus sunitinib alone. Sunitinib alone was found noninferior to combination therapy. The median overall survival in the sunitinib-only group was 18.4 months (14.7–23.0 mo) in comparison to 13.9 months (11.8–18.3 mo) in patients receiving CN followed by sunitinib. Although the study was not powered for a subgroup analysis, MSKCC intermediate-

risk patients' median overall survival was 23.4 months in sunitinib-only versus 19.0 months with combination therapy, and 13.3 months versus 10.2 months, respectively, in poor-risk patients.[52]

Several important conclusions can be drawn from CARMENA. First, patient selection for CN is vital and CN should not be considered standard of care for all-comers with mRCC. Patients with intermediate-risk and poor-risk disease should not undergo CN routinely when systemic medical treatment is required or if it would not improve quality of life.[53] CARMENA included patients who were not expected to benefit from CN based on retrospective studies, with 43% of patients having poor-risk disease and high metastatic burden, explaining why overall survival was lower in CARMENA than in other recent trials. CARMENA further supported that CN not only is ineffective but also may be harmful in patients with poor-risk mRCC.[43] Second, CARMENA highlights that not all patients who undergo CN will receive systemic therapy, the mainstay of metastatic treatment. In this trial, 17.7% of patients in the combination arm did not receive sunitinib after CN. Lastly, some patients with intermediate-risk and poor-risk disease may benefit from CN by reducing adverse events and improving quality of life. The CN group had fewer grade 3 and grade 4 adverse events (32.8% vs 42.7%, respectively), which included significantly fewer renal or urinary tract disorders (0.5% vs 4.2%, respectively), anemia, and musculoskeletal disorders; 17% of patients in the sunitinib-only arm underwent secondary CN for symptomatic management or in cases of complete or near-complete response.[52] CN may be used palliatively to improve symptoms caused by the primary renal tumor and overall quality of life.

CARMENA helped clarify management of MSKCC intermediate-risk and poor-risk mRCC, but it does not provide guidance for favorable-risk patients. The Targeted Therapy With or Without Nephrectomy in Metastatic Renal Cell Carcinoma: Liquid Biopsy dor Biomarkers Discovery (TARIBO) trial was a similarly designed trial comparing CN with TKI to TKI alone and included MSKCC favorable-risk and intermediate-risk patients. Unfortunately, the trial was terminated due to low recruitment, a common problem in many mRCC trials, leading to underpowered data or trial termination.[54]

A second RCT, Immediate Surgery or Surgery After Sunitinib Malate in Treating Patients With Metastatic Kidney Cancer (SURTIME) explored the timing of CN in relation to initiation of systemic VEGF-TKI therapy in patients with metastatic disease (see **Table 1**).[55] SURTIME compared predominantly MSKCC intermediate-risk patients (88% intermediate risk and 12% poor risk) receiving upfront CN followed by sunitinib to 3 cycles of sunitinib followed by CN with continued sunitinib. It attempted to determine if delayed CN would improve outcomes in comparison to immediate CN and if presurgical systemic therapy could help select patients who would benefit from surgery. Unfortunately, the trial was underpowered, enrolling 99 patients from an anticipated 458 patients, partly due to strict eligibility criteria, including only the best surgical candidates. The primary endpoint of progression-free survival was not met, but an exploratory secondary endpoint of overall survival substantially favored the deferred CN arm on intent-to-treat analysis with a median overall survival of 32.4 months versus 15.1 months respectively ($P = .032$) and an HR of 0.57 (95% CI, 0.34–0.95).[55,56] Despite the studies' limitations, the data support the conclusions drawn from CARMENA that delaying systemic therapy for immediate CN in patients with intermediate-risk and poor-risk disease decreases survival and systemic therapy is the most important treatment component in improving patient outcomes with mRCC. It remains unclear whether intermediate-risk patients who have stable or regressive disease on initial systemic VEGF-TKI therapy would receive additional benefit from undergoing deferred CN.[53]

ACTIVE SURVEILLANCE

Metastatic RCC is characterized by diverse biology and wide-ranging natural history. The prospective trials from the VEGF-TKI era fail to elucidate the possible benefits of CN in patients with good performance status, low-volume metastatic disease, and favorable risk or intermediate risk who may not require systemic therapy. In 2016, a phase II trial evaluated patients with mRCC using an active surveillance protocol, waiting for evidence of progression to initiate systemic therapy.[57] All patients were MSKCC favorable risk or intermediate risk, 98% had undergone prior nephrectomy, and median time on active surveillance until systemic therapy initiation was 14.9 months. A favorable-risk subset, defined by few IMDC risk criteria and at most 2 metastatic sites, had a median surveillance time of 22 months versus 8.4 months in the unfavorable-risk subset.[57] This study emphasizes not all patients with mRCC require immediate systemic therapy and that patients with favorable-risk, low-volume disease, who undergo nephrectomy or CN, may benefit from a substantial period free from toxic systemic treatment.

NEW ERA—IMMUNO-ONCOLOGY

The development of VEGF-TKI therapy altered the treatment paradigm of mRCC, highlighting the importance of systemic treatment in improving outcomes in patients with intermediate-risk and poor-risk disease. A new transition is under way with immune-oncology (IO) checkpoint inhibitors. The landmark CheckMate 214 study published in 2018 was a phase III RCT comparing combination ipilimumab and nivolumab (ipi-nivo) to sunitinib in patients with mostly IMDC intermediate-risk and poor-risk disease (see **Table 1**).[58,59] Patients receiving checkpoint inhibition had superior outcomes to those receiving VEGF-TKI in 18-month overall survival rate (75% vs 60%, respectively), median overall survival (not reached vs 26.6 mo, respectively), objective response rate (42% vs 29%, respectively; $P < .001$), complete response (11% vs 2%, respectively), and grade 3 or grade 4 adverse events (46% vs 63%, respectively).[58,59]

Following CheckMate 214, ipi-nivo replaced sunitinib as first-line treatment of intermediate-risk and poor-risk mRCC.

New trials are under way to evaluate combinations of IO and VEGF-targeted therapy (IOVE) to further advance systemic treatments.[60] IOVE therapy has universally demonstrated improved response rates and progression-free survival in direct comparison over sunitinib monotherapy, and the combination of axitinib plus pembrolizumab additionally has demonstrated improved overall survival (see **Table 1**).[61–63] In comparing IOVE to ipi-nivo, a recent retrospective review found no significant differences in first-line outcomes, such as time to treatment failure, but suggested a greater response to second-line VEGF-based therapy when ipi-nivo was used as the first-line treatment.[64] New prospective studies are needed to determine optimal systemic treatment of each mRCC risk group.

Implementing immune checkpoint inhibitors into the treatment of mRCC has renewed excitement through the observation of complete responses and improved prognosis. In addition to determining the most efficacious IO combination, trials are needed to re-evaluate the role of CN with these more potent therapies.

CYTOREDUCTIVE NEPHRECTOMY IN METASTATIC NON–CLEAR CELL METASTATIC RENAL CELL CARCINOMA

Limited data exist evaluating CN in patients with non–clear cell mRCC. The landmark studies of the cytokine and targeted therapy eras, including SWOG 8949, EORTC 30947, CARMENA, and SURTIME, all excluded patients with non–clear cell histology. Several retrospective series have demonstrated favorable outcomes with CN in non–clear cell mRCC, but these trials are fraught with bias. A retrospective analysis of the SEER database from 2001 to 2014 included 851 patients with non–clear cell mRCC and showed that patients who underwent CN had a 2-year mortality rate of 52.6% in comparison to 77.8% in the group that did not receive CN.[65] A similar analysis of the IMDC database for 353 patients with synchronous papillary mRCC treated with targeted therapy with or without CN found a median overall survival advantage in the CN group of 16.3 months versus 8.6 months, respectively.[66] Overall, CN appears to improve survival in patients with non–clear cell mRCC based on retrospective data from the targeted therapy era. As learned from CARMENA and SURTIME, the favorable outcomes seen in retrospective series may not persist with more rigorous RCTs. Prospective trials are needed to evaluate the role of CN in patients with non–clear cell mRCC, particularly in the IO/IOVE era, to determine its efficacy.

EUROPEAN ASSOCIATION OF UROLOGY RECOMMENDATIONS AND NATIONAL COMPREHENSIVE CANCER NETWORK GUIDELINES

In August 2018, the European Association of Urology (EAU) updated guidelines for CN in patients with synchronous metastatic clear cell RCC based on the results of the recent prospective RCTs evaluating the role of CN with VEGF-TKsI systemic therapy. In their statements, the EAU strongly recommends against the use of CN in MSKCC poor-risk patients. In MSKCC intermediate-risk disease, they recommend systemic therapy. They recommend against performing immediate CN but suggest discussing delayed CN in patients who derive long-term sustained benefit and/or minimal residual metastatic burden on VEGF-TKI therapy. Immediate CN is recommended only in patients with good performance status and who do not require immediate-risk systemic therapy.[53]

The EAU and National Comprehensive Cancer Network (NCCN) guidelines for management of metastatic disease with systemic therapy reflect emerging data. In the 2019 update, the EAU recommends pembrolizumab plus axitinib (IOVE) for IMDC favorable-risk, intermediate-risk, and poor-risk disease or ipi-nivo for intermediate-risk and poor-risk disease as first-line therapy.[67] Similarly, NCCN guidelines recommend axitinib plus pembrolizumab followed by sunitinib or pazopanib as first line for favorable-risk clear cell RCC and ipi-nivo followed by axitinib plus pembrolizumab or cabozantinib as first line for intermediate-risk or poor-risk disease. In non–clear cell histology, NCCN recommends sunitinib or a clinical trial as first-line systemic therapy.[13] Current guidelines have not been updated to reflect the role for CN in the IO and IOVE era due to lack of trials and evidence.

TAKE-HOME POINTS AND CLINICAL RECOMMENDATIONS

Advancements in systemic therapy have altered how surgical management should be utilized in patients with mRCC. Although CN was once standard of care during the cytokine-based immunotherapy era, it no longer should be offered to all-comers with systemic disease. CN offers a survival advantage only when thoughtfully combined with systemic therapy. Unfortunately, upfront CN leads to a delay in initiation of systemic treatment and not all patients who undergo CN may be able to receive systemic therapy. This delay likely explains why CN may be harmful to patients with more advanced metastatic disease and highlights the importance of systemic therapy. Results from CARMENA and SURTIME suggest that MSKCC intermediate-risk and poor-risk disease patients have worse outcomes when they undergo upfront CN in comparison to delayed CN or VEGF-TKI monotherapy. In general, patients with poor risk disease and most with intermediate risk disease need immediate systemic therapy and should not undergo upfront CN. IO and IOVE therapy are now surpassing VEGF-TKI therapy as first-line treatments of mRCC.

CN may still be beneficial when limited to specific mRCC patient populations. First, patients with good performance status, low-volume, favorable-risk mRCC may have a survival advantage with CN, although level 1 evidence does not exist. Second, CN still may be appropriate in patients who do not require urgent systemic therapy. Patients who can be observed without immediate initiation of systemic therapy can proceed with CN and then be followed on an active surveillance protocol, possibly benefiting from a substantial delay in initiation of toxic systemic treatment. Third, patients with favorable-risk or intermediate-risk mRCC who respond to systemic therapy, with stable or regressive disease, may consider delayed CN. In this capacity, response to systemic therapy could serve as a litmus test for selecting appropriate patients for CN. Fourth, CN may be offered to patients with symptomatic mRCC to improve quality of life. Overall, CN in the modern IO/IOVE era requires further evaluation to identify which mRCC patient populations may still receive benefit from CN, and to understand how CN should be optimally timed with systemic therapy.

CONFLICTS OF INTEREST

None.

REFERENCES

1. Institue NC. Cancer stat facts: kidney and renal pelvis cancer. SEER Database 2019.
2. Patel HD, Gupta M, Joice GA, et al. Clinical stage migration and survival for renal cell carcinoma in the United States. Eur Urol Oncol 2019;2:343–8.
3. Kane CJ, Mallin K, Ritchey J, et al. Renal cell cancer stage migration: analysis of the National Cancer Data Base. Cancer 2008;113:78–83.
4. Lam JS, Shvarts O, Leppert JT, et al. Renal cell carcinoma 2005: new frontiers in staging, prognostication and targeted molecular therapy. J Urol 2005; 173:1853–62.
5. Thorstenson A, Bergman M, Scherman-Plogell AH, et al. Tumour characteristics and surgical treatment of renal cell carcinoma in Sweden 2005-2010: a population-based study from the national Swedish kidney cancer register. Scand J Urol 2014;48:231–8.
6. Ball MW. Surgical management of metastatic renal cell carcinoma. Discov Med 2017;23:379–87.
7. Motzer RJ, Hutson TE, Tomczak P, et al. Sunitinib versus interferon alfa in metastatic renal-cell carcinoma. N Engl J Med 2007;356:115–24.
8. Pindoria N, Raison N, Blecher G, et al. Cytoreductive nephrectomy in the era of targeted therapies: a review. BJU Int 2017;120:320–8.
9. Negrier S, Escudier B, Gomez F, et al. Prognostic factors of survival and rapid progression in 782 patients with metastatic renal carcinomas treated by cytokines: a report from the Groupe Francais d'Immunotherapie. Ann Oncol 2002;13:1460–8.
10. Motzer RJ, Russo P. Systemic therapy for renal cell carcinoma. J Urol 2000;163:408–17.
11. Motzer RJ, Mazumdar M, Bacik J, et al. Survival and prognostic stratification of 670 patients with advanced renal cell carcinoma. J Clin Oncol 1999; 17:2530–40.
12. Escudier B, Porta C, Schmidinger M, et al. Renal cell carcinoma: ESMO clinical practice guidelines for diagnosis, treatment and follow-up. Ann Oncol 2016;27:v58–68.
13. Motzer RJ, Jonasch E, Agarwal N, et al. Kidney cancer, version 2.2017, NCCN clinical practice guidelines in oncology. J Natl Compr Canc Netw 2017; 15:804–34.
14. Flanigan RC, Salmon SE, Blumenstein BA, et al. Nephrectomy followed by interferon alfa-2b compared with interferon alfa-2b alone for metastatic renal-cell cancer. N Engl J Med 2001;345:1655–9.
15. Mickisch GH, Garin A, van Poppel H, et al. Radical nephrectomy plus interferon-alfa-based immunotherapy compared with interferon alfa alone in metastatic renal-cell carcinoma: a randomised trial. Lancet 2001;358:966–70.
16. Flanigan RC, Mickisch G, Sylvester R, et al. Cytoreductive nephrectomy in patients with metastatic renal cancer: a combined analysis. J Urol 2004; 171:1071–6.
17. Turajlic S, Xu H, Litchfield K, et al. Tracking cancer evolution reveals constrained routes to metastases: TRACERx renal. Cell 2018;173:581–94.e12.
18. Marcus SG, Choyke PL, Reiter R, et al. Regression of metastatic renal cell carcinoma after cytoreductive nephrectomy. J Urol 1993;150:463–6.
19. Garfield DH, Kennedy BJ. Regression of metastatic renal cell carcinoma following nephrectomy. Cancer 1972;30:190–6.
20. Chery LJ, Karam JA, Wood CG. Cytoreductive nephrectomy for metastatic renal cell carcinoma. Clin Adv Hematol Oncol 2016;14:696–703.

21. Uzzo RG, Clark PE, Rayman P, et al. Alterations in NFkappaB activation in T lymphocytes of patients with renal cell carcinoma. J Natl Cancer Inst 1999; 91:718–21.

22. Ling W, Rayman P, Uzzo R, et al. Impaired activation of NFkappaB in T cells from a subset of renal cell carcinoma patients is mediated by inhibition of phosphorylation and degradation of the inhibitor, IkappaBalpha. Blood 1998;92:1334–41.

23. Remark R, Alifano M, Cremer I, et al. Characteristics and clinical impacts of the immune environments in colorectal and renal cell carcinoma lung metastases: influence of tumor origin. Clin Cancer Res 2013;19:4079–91.

24. Perut F, Cenni E, Unger RE, et al. Immunogenic properties of renal cell carcinoma and the pathogenesis of osteolytic bone metastases. Int J Oncol 2009; 34:1387–93.

25. Williams T, Rodriguez R, Murray K, et al. Metastatic papillary renal cell carcinoma regression after cytoreductive nephrectomy. Urology 2015;85:283–7.

26. Fyfe G, Fisher RI, Rosenberg SA, et al. Results of treatment of 255 patients with metastatic renal cell carcinoma who received high-dose recombinant interleukin-2 therapy. J Clin Oncol 1995;13: 688–96.

27. Heng DY, Xie W, Regan MM, et al. Prognostic factors for overall survival in patients with metastatic renal cell carcinoma treated with vascular endothelial growth factor-targeted agents: results from a large, multicenter study. J Clin Oncol 2009;27: 5794–9.

28. Heng DY, Xie W, Regan MM, et al. External validation and comparison with other models of the International Metastatic Renal-Cell Carcinoma Database Consortium prognostic model: a population-based study. Lancet Oncol 2013;14:141–8.

29. Culp SH, Tannir NM, Abel EJ, et al. Can we better select patients with metastatic renal cell carcinoma for cytoreductive nephrectomy? Cancer 2010;116: 3378–88.

30. Fallick ML, McDermott DF, LaRock D, et al. Nephrectomy before interleukin-2 therapy for patients with metastatic renal cell carcinoma. J Urol 1997;158: 1691–5.

31. Leibovich BC, Han KR, Bui MH, et al. Scoring algorithm to predict survival after nephrectomy and immunotherapy in patients with metastatic renal cell carcinoma: a stratification tool for prospective clinical trials. Cancer 2003;98:2566–75.

32. Patel HD, Gorin MA, Gupta N, et al. Mortality trends and the impact of lymphadenectomy on survival for renal cell carcinoma patients with distant metastasis. Can Urol Assoc J 2016;10:389–95.

33. Ohno Y, Nakashima J, Ohori M, et al. Clinical variables for predicting metastatic renal cell carcinoma patients who might not benefit from cytoreductive nephrectomy: neutrophil-to-lymphocyte ratio and performance status. Int J Clin Oncol 2014;19: 139–45.

34. Sharma P, Zargar-Shoshtari K, Caracciolo JT, et al. Sarcopenia as a predictor of overall survival after cytoreductive nephrectomy for metastatic renal cell carcinoma. Urol Oncol 2015;33:339.e17-23.

35. Corcoran AT, Kaffenberger SD, Clark PE, et al. Hypoalbuminaemia is associated with mortality in patients undergoing cytoreductive nephrectomy. BJU Int 2015;116:351–7.

36. Hudes G, Carducci M, Tomczak P, et al. Temsirolimus, interferon alfa, or both for advanced renal-cell carcinoma. N Engl J Med 2007;356:2271–81.

37. Escudier B, Eisen T, Stadler WM, et al. Sorafenib in advanced clear-cell renal-cell carcinoma. N Engl J Med 2007;356:125–34.

38. Patel HD, Karam JA, Allaf ME. Surgical management of advanced kidney cancer: the role of cytoreductive nephrectomy and lymphadenectomy. Journal of Clinical Oncology 2018 36;36:3601–7.

39. Shah AY, Karam JA, Lim ZD, et al. Clinical and pathological complete remission in a patient with metastatic renal cell carcinoma (mRCC) treated with sunitinib: Is mRCC curable with targeted therapy? Urol Case Rep 2015;3:18–20.

40. Psutka SP, Kim SP, Gross CP, et al. The impact of targeted therapy on management of metastatic renal cell carcinoma: trends in systemic therapy and cytoreductive nephrectomy utilization. Urology 2015;85: 442–50.

41. Choueiri TK, Xie W, Kollmannsberger C, et al. The impact of cytoreductive nephrectomy on survival of patients with metastatic renal cell carcinoma receiving vascular endothelial growth factor targeted therapy. J Urol 2011;185:60–6.

42. Conti SL, Thomas IC, Hagedorn JC, et al. Utilization of cytoreductive nephrectomy and patient survival in the targeted therapy era. Int J Cancer 2014;134: 2245–52.

43. Heng DY, Wells JC, Rini BI, et al. Cytoreductive nephrectomy in patients with synchronous metastases from renal cell carcinoma: results from the International Metastatic Renal Cell Carcinoma Database Consortium. Eur Urol 2014;66:704–10.

44. Bamias A, Tzannis K, Papatsoris A, et al. Prognostic significance of cytoreductive nephrectomy in patients with synchronous metastases from renal cell carcinoma treated with first-line sunitinib: a European multiinstitutional study. Clin Genitourin Cancer 2014;12:373–83.

45. Abern MR, Scosyrev E, Tsivian M, et al. Survival of patients undergoing cytoreductive surgery for metastatic renal cell carcinoma in the targeted-therapy era. Anticancer Res 2014;34:2405–11.

46. Aizer AA, Urun Y, McKay RR, et al. Cytoreductive nephrectomy in patients with metastatic non-clear-cell

renal cell carcinoma (RCC). BJU Int 2014;113: E67–74.

47. Mathieu R, Pignot G, Ingles A, et al. Nephrectomy improves overall survival in patients with metastatic renal cell carcinoma in cases of favorable MSKCC or ECOG prognostic features. Urol Oncol 2015;33: 339.e9-15.

48. de Groot S, Redekop WK, Sleijfer S, et al. Survival in patients with primary metastatic renal cell carcinoma treated with sunitinib with or without previous cytoreductive nephrectomy: results from a population-based registry. Urology 2016;95:121–7.

49. Hanna N, Sun M, Meyer CP, et al. Survival analyses of patients with metastatic renal cancer treated with targeted therapy with or without cytoreductive nephrectomy: a national cancer data base study. J Clin Oncol 2016;34:3267–75.

50. Petrelli F, Coinu A, Vavassori I, et al. Cytoreductive nephrectomy in metastatic renal cell carcinoma treated with targeted therapies: a systematic review with a meta-analysis. Clin Genitourin Cancer 2016; 14:465–72.

51. Bex A, Ljungberg B, van Poppel H, et al. The role of cytoreductive nephrectomy: European Association of Urology Recommendations in 2016. Eur Urol 2016;70:901–5.

52. Mejean A, Ravaud A, Thezenas S, et al. Sunitinib alone or after nephrectomy in metastatic renal-cell carcinoma. N Engl J Med 2018;379:417–27.

53. Bex A, Albiges L, Ljungberg B, et al. Updated European Association of Urology Guidelines for cytoreductive nephrectomy in patients with synchronous metastatic clear-cell renal cell carcinoma. Eur Urol 2018;74:805–9.

54. Verzoni E, Ratta R, Grassi P, et al. TARIBO trial: targeted therapy with or without nephrectomy in metastatic renal cell carcinoma: liquid biopsy for biomarkers discovery. Tumori 2018;104:401–5.

55. Bex A, Mulders P, Jewett M, et al. Comparison of immediate vs deferred cytoreductive nephrectomy in patients with synchronous metastatic renal cell carcinoma receiving sunitinib: The SURTIME randomized clinical trial. JAMA Oncol 2019;5:164–70.

56. De Bruijn RE, Mulders P, Jewett MA, et al. Surgical safety of cytoreductive nephrectomy following sunitinib: results from the multicentre, randomised controlled trial of immediate versus deferred nephrectomy (SURTIME). Eur Urol 2019;76:437–40.

57. Rini BI, Dorff TB, Elson P, et al. Active surveillance in metastatic renal-cell carcinoma: a prospective, phase 2 trial. Lancet Oncol 2016;17:1317–24.

58. Motzer RJ, Tannir NM, McDermott DF, et al. Nivolumab plus ipilimumab versus sunitinib in advanced renal-cell carcinoma. N Engl J Med 2018;378: 1277–90.

59. Motzer RJ, Rini BI, McDermott DF, et al. Nivolumab plus ipilimumab versus sunitinib in first-line treatment for advanced renal cell carcinoma: extended follow-up of efficacy and safety results from a randomised, controlled, phase 3 trial. Lancet Oncol 2019;20:1370–85.

60. Lalani AA, McGregor BA, Albiges L, et al. Systemic treatment of metastatic clear cell renal cell carcinoma in 2018: current paradigms, use of immunotherapy, and future directions. Eur Urol 2019;75: 100–10.

61. Rini BI, Powles T, Atkins MB, et al. Atezolizumab plus bevacizumab versus sunitinib in patients with previously untreated metastatic renal cell carcinoma (IMmotion151): a multicentre, open-label, phase 3, randomised controlled trial. Lancet 2019;393: 2404–15.

62. Motzer RJ, Penkov K, Haanen J, et al. Avelumab plus axitinib versus sunitinib for advanced renal-cell carcinoma. N Engl J Med 2019;380:1103–15.

63. Rini BI, Plimack ER, Stus V, et al. Pembrolizumab plus axitinib versus sunitinib for advanced renal-cell carcinoma. N Engl J Med 2019;380: 1116–27.

64. Dudani S, Graham J, Wells JC, et al. First-line immuno-oncology combination therapies in metastatic renal-cell carcinoma: results from the international metastatic renal-cell carcinoma database consortium. Eur Urol 2019;76:861–7.

65. Marchioni M, Bandini M, Preisser F, et al. Survival after cytoreductive nephrectomy in metastatic non-clear cell renal cell carcinoma patients: a population-based study. Eur Urol Focus 2019;5: 488–96.

66. Graham J, Wells JC, Donskov F, et al. Cytoreductive nephrectomy in metastatic papillary renal cell carcinoma: results from the international metastatic renal cell carcinoma database consortium. Eur Urol Oncol 2019;2:643–8.

67. Albiges L, Powles T, Staehler M, et al. Updated European Association of urology guidelines on renal cell carcinoma: immune checkpoint inhibition is the new backbone in first-line treatment of metastatic clear-cell renal cell carcinoma. Eur Urol 2019;76: 151–6.

The Role of Lymphadenectomy in Patients with Advanced Renal Cell Carcinoma

Pooja Unadkat, MD, Aria F. Olumi, MD, Boris Gershman, MD*

KEYWORDS

- Renal cell carcinoma • Lymph node dissection • Template • Indications • Survival • Outcomes

KEY POINTS

- Lymph node dissection serves an important staging role by providing pathologic lymph node stage, which has been independently associated with survival in nonmetastatic and metastatic renal cell carcinoma.
- Lymph node dissection does not seem to provide a survival benefit for nonmetastatic or metastatic renal cell carcinoma, even in patients at increased risk for lymph node metastases.
- Most patients with clinically isolated lymph node involvement develop systemic progression within the first year after surgery, although a small subset demonstrates long-term recurrence-free survival.
- Lymph node dissection is not associated with an increased risk of perioperative morbidity when performed in experienced centers.

INTRODUCTION AND HISTORICAL PERSPECTIVE

Lymph node dissection (LND) plays a central role in the management of urologic malignancies. However, its role in the management of renal cell carcinoma (RCC) has been controversial.[1–4] Although LND provides indisputable pathologic nodal staging, its impact on survival has been uncertain. The attribution of a potential survival benefit to LND can be traced back to Robson's seminal description of radical nephrectomy in 1969, wherein the authors suggested that the improved survival of patients in that series, compared to contemporaneous reports, was due in part to the performance of a thorough lympadenectomy.[5]

Since then, a number of observational studies have similarly suggested improved survival with LND.[6–8] However, the only randomized trial to examine this question, EORTC 30881, reported no survival benefit upon its publication in 2009.[9] Despite criticism that the trial enrolled overwhelmingly low-risk patients, and that LND may still benefit those at higher risk of lymph node metastases, more recent investigations have not supported a therapeutic benefit to LND, even in locally advanced or metastatic RCC.[1,10–15] Still, LND provides valuable prognostic data, and as such may have a role for improved staging.

In this article, we review the contemporary role of LND in the management of locally advanced and metastatic RCC. We critically evaluate the available evidence base to address several important clinical questions, including the indications for LND, optimal LND templates, staging role, survival benefit, and morbidity.

LYMPH NODE DISSECTION TEMPLATES

To examine the role of LND, it is essential to first define the templates and techniques for LND. In

Division of Urologic Surgery, Beth Israel Deaconess Medical Center, Boston, MA 02215, USA
* Corresponding author.
E-mail address: bgershma@bidmc.harvard.edu

Urol Clin N Am 47 (2020) 371–377
https://doi.org/10.1016/j.ucl.2020.04.001
0094-0143/20/© 2020 Elsevier Inc. All rights reserved.

contrast with retroperitoneal LND for testicular cancer[16] or pelvic LND for prostate cancer,[17] there is no standardized, universally accepted template or templates for performing LND for RCC.[18–20] However, several principles for LND can be inferred based on both anatomic and clinical studies.[21–23]

The anatomic basis for retroperitoneal lymphatic drainage has been described in several anatomic studies.[21] Such studies demonstrate renal lymphatic drainage into the retroperitoneal lymph nodes, with side-specific preferential drainage of the right kidney into the hilar, pre-caval, and interaortocaval lymph nodes, whereas the left kidney drains into the hilar, para-aortic, and interaortocaval lymph nodes.[21] However, drainage patterns vary tremendously, and direct communication of the efferent lymphatics to the thoracic duct have also been described. Further complicating these heterogeneous drainage patterns, direct lymphovenous communications to the renal vein and vena cava have been reported, likewise bypassing the retroperitoneal lymph nodes altogether.[21]

More recently, an in vivo study using sentinel lymph node mapping with single photon emission computed tomography reinforced the unpredictable lymphatic drainage pattern of RCC and the potential for bypassing the retroperitoneal lymph nodes.[22] In that study, 35% of patients were found to have sentinel lymphatic drainage outside the locoregional retroperitoneal template, including 20% for whom sentinel nodes were supradiaphragmatic.[22] Such data reinforce the overarching concept that lymphatic drainage for RCC does not follow a uniform, step-wise drainage pattern, an understanding that has important implications for the role of lymphadenectomy.

Few clinical studies have examined the optimal template for LND. In a seminal study, Crispen and colleagues[23] characterized patterns of lymphatic spread in 169 patients at high risk for lymph node metastases. They reported the notable observation that there were no skip metastases to the contralateral lymph nodes without involvement of the interaortocaval lymph nodes: for right-sided tumors, there was no involvement of para-aortic lymph nodes without interaortocaval involvement; and for left-sided tumors, there was no involvement of para-caval lymph nodes without interaortocaval involvement (**Fig. 1**). Based on these observations, the authors recommended that patients without clinical lymphadenopathy undergo removal of the lymph nodes surrounding the ipsilateral great vessel to the interaortocaval lymph nodes, from the crus of the diaphragm to the common iliac arteries; if the interaortocaval lymph nodes are positive, then a full bilateral dissection should be performed.[23]

Furthermore, there are data to support the logical concept that a more extensive LND is associated with better staging accuracy. For instance, Terrone and colleagues[24] noted that a more extensive lymphadenectomy was associated with increased detection of lymph node metastases, suggesting at least 13 lymph nodes be removed for adequate staging. Several other studies have also suggested that a more extended LND may be associated with improved survival, although these findings must be reconciled within the overall body of evidence suggesting no benefit to LND (discussed in detail elsewhere in this article).[7,25]

STAGING ROLE OF LYMPH NODE DISSECTION

Radiographic staging has poor performance for the identification of lymph node metastases from RCC.[26–29] Although the classical 1-cm size threshold for radiographically enlarged lymph nodes is quite specific for the diagnosis of metastatic disease in other urologic malignancies such as prostate or bladder cancers, radiographic lymphadenopathy has poor specificity in RCC.[29] For instance, in a seminal study by Studer and colleagues,[29] the authors reported that only 42% of patients with radiographically enlarged lymph nodes on computed tomography harbored pathologically confirmed RCC, while 58% of these patients were found to have only inflammatory changes. A more recent investigation reinforced these findings, reporting that there was an approximately linear relationship between lymph node short axis diameter and the risk of pN1 disease.[30] In that study, the risk of lymph node metastases ranged from approximately 29% for 1.0 cm short axis diameter to 90% at 3.0 cm.[30] Conversely, cross-sectional imaging is relatively good for excluding lymph node metastases; for instance, only 4.4% of patients with cN0 disease in the EORTC 30881 trial had occult lymph node metastases,[9] similar to the 3.1% false-negative rate for computed tomography in the study by Studer and colleagues.[29]

Given the poor performance of radiographic imaging for the identification of lymph node metastases, several groups have developed predictive models for pN1 disease.[1] For instance, Blute and colleagues[23,31] reported that tumor size greater than 10 cm, stage pT3/T4, nuclear grade 3 to 4, and presence of coagulative tumor necrosis or sarcomatoid differentiation were associated with pN1 disease, validating these findings in a prospective investigation. Other groups have developed nomograms to predict the risk of pN1

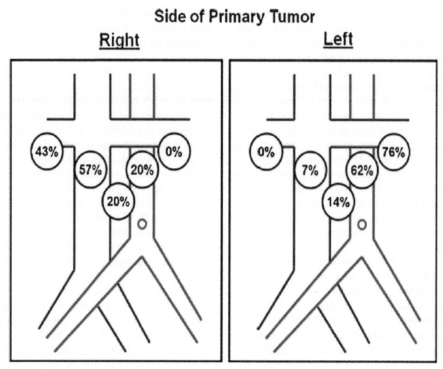

Fig. 1. Location of positive lymph nodes based on side of primary tumor. Reported percentage represents frequency of involved location in patients with lymph node–positive disease. (*From* Crispen PL, Breau RH, Allmer C, et al. Lymph node dissection at the time of radical nephrectomy for high-risk clear cell renal cell carcinoma: indications and recommendations for surgical templates. Eur Urol. 2011;59(1):18-23; with permission.)

disease, identifying similar clinicopathologic features as being associated with lymph node metastases.[32–34]

Despite the availability of clinical risk prediction models to identify patients with pN1 disease, there is no substitute for pathologic lymph node staging. Indeed, LND serves as the gold standard in establishing nodal stage. Accordingly, it provides actionable data to improve prognostication and guide postoperative management. For instance, it may identify patients for consideration of adjuvant systemic therapy after surgery, enrollment into clinical trials, or the use of more intensive surveillance imaging.[1]

Nodal stage provides valuable prognostic information.[1] Multiple studies have reported that, even when adjusting for other clinicopathologic features, both clinical nodal (cN) stage and pathologic nodal (pN) stage are independently associated with survival.[1,11,35–37] Remarkably, nodal stage remains prognostic even in the setting of metastatic RCC. Although it may seem logical that the presence of distant metastatic disease should drive prognosis regardless of the presence of nodal metastases, several studies have reported that lymph node metastases are associated with more

aggressive tumor biology, even in the M1 setting.[12,37] For instance, pN1 tumors have an increased incidence of higher pT stage, coagulative tumor necrosis, and sarcomatoid differentiation.[12,37] These findings may explain why lymph node metastases carry an adverse prognosis, even in the setting of metastatic RCC.

SURVIVAL BENEFIT OF LYMPH NODE DISSECTION IN M0 RENAL CELL CARCINOMA

The question of whether LND confers a survival benefit has generated interest for more than 50 years, dating back to the original description of radical nephrectomy by Robson and co-workers.[5] However, although a number of studies have examined this topic,[6–8] there were few high-quality data to inform clinical practice until recent years. The highest level of evidence has been provided by the only randomized trial to examine LND in RCC, EORTC 30881.[9] In that study, 772 patients with cT1 to 3 cN0 cM0 RCC were randomized to radical nephrectomy with LND or radical nephrectomy alone. At a median follow-up of 12.6 years, there was no statistically significant difference in any oncologic end point examined, including disease progression or death.[9] It is important to underscore that the study population had a low incidence of lymph node metastases of only 4.0%.

More recently conducted observational studies, as well as a meta-analysis of such studies, have similarly reported no survival benefit in M0 patients at average risk of lymph node metastases (Fig. 2).[1,10,13,14] In a meta-analysis of EORTC 30881 and 3 observational studies with multivariable statistical adjustment, the pooled hazard ratio for the association of LND with survival was 1.02 and not statistically significant (95% confidence interval, 0.92–1.12). Thus, both randomized and high-quality observational data agree that LND does not confer a survival benefit in average-risk patients with clinically localized, node-negative (cN0) RCC.

Because removal of benign lymph nodes cannot be expected to improve survival, it is logical to examine whether LND may confer a survival advantage in patients at higher risk of lymph node metastases. Support for this concept was provided by an older observational study, in which the authors reported improved survival for cN1 patients who underwent LND compared with patients who did not.[6] However, methodologic limitations in that study (eg, multivariable adjustment limited to only 5 variables) limit causal inference from these results.

Several more recent studies have also examined the survival benefit of LND in higher risk patients. In one institutional study of 1797 patients with M0 RCC, the authors examined two high-risk patient subsets: patients with cN1 RCC and patients stratified by predicted probability of pN1 disease ranging from ≥10% to ≥50%.[13] In both high-risk subsets, LND was not associated with a decreased risk of distant metastases, cancer-specific mortality, or all-cause mortality. In another study in which the authors conducted a secondary analysis of the ASSURE (ECOG-ACRIN 2805) trial, there was no difference in disease-free or overall survival.[14] Notably, this was a high-risk population by design, because the trial enrolled patients with grade 3 to 4 pT1b N0, pT2 to 4 N0, or pTany N+ RCC, and is reflected in a pN+ rate of 23.4%. In a third study, in which the authors conducted a secondary analysis of EORTC 30881, examining patients with cT3 tumors, there was no statistically significant difference in overall survival.[15] It is worth noting that, even when considering a seemingly higher risk cohort of patients with cT3 tumors, the rate of lymph node metastases was still only 6.3%.[15] Taken together, these studies suggest that there is no survival benefit to LND in cN1 RCC or in otherwise high-risk patients for lymph node metastases.

These discrepancies between the underlying biologic plausibility for a survival benefit to LND and the lack thereof in published studies may be reconciled by considering the anatomic basis for lymphatic drainage in RCC, as well as the tumor characteristics of lymph node positive disease. As discussed elsewhere in this article, renal

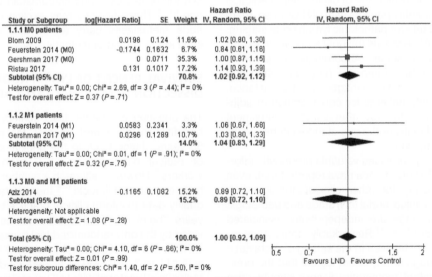

Fig. 2. Forest plot for meta-analysis of the association of LND with oncologic outcomes among patients with M0 and M1 disease. (*From* Bhindi B, Wallis CJD, Boorjian SA, et al. The role of lymph node dissection in the management of renal cell carcinoma: a systematic review and meta-analysis. *BJU international*. 2018;121(5):684-698; with permission.)

lymphatic drainage may frequently bypass retroperitoneal lymph nodes, with early hematogenous dissemination from direct lymphovenous communications or nonretroperitoneal sentinel lymphatic drainage.[21,22] Moreover, the presence of lymph node metastases is associated with more aggressive tumor biology, such as higher pT stage, coagulative tumor necrosis, and sarcomatoid differentiation.[12,37]

SURVIVAL BENEFIT OF LYMPH NODE DISSECTION IN M1 RENAL CELL CARCINOMA

The underlying biologic plausibility for a survival benefit to LND in the metastatic setting borrows from cytoreductive principles in kidney cancer. For instance, two randomized trials conducted in the immunotherapy era demonstrated that, in properly selected patients, cytoreductive nephrectomy followed by interferon-alpha was associated with improved survival compared with interferon-alpha alone.[38,39] Such trials support the hypothesis that cytoreductive surgery may decrease the tumor burden, alleviate tumor-mediated immunosuppression, and improve the response to systemic therapy.

Few high-quality studies have examined the survival benefit of LND in M1 RCC.[1] In one institutional analysis of 305 patients who underwent cytoreductive nephrectomy, including 62% with concomitant LND, LND was not associated with a difference in cancer-specific or all-cause mortality.[12] Moreover, there was no survival benefit to LND, even among patients with cN1 RCC or across increasing probability thresholds for pN1 disease, ranging from 20% to 80%. In another study of 258 patients undergoing cytoreductive nephrectomy, including 69% who underwent LND, there was no difference in overall survival.[11]

Despite the underlying biologic plausibility discussed elsewhere in this article, the lack of a survival benefit to LND in the metastatic setting likely reflects the finding that lymph node–positive disease is more often associated with aggressive disease biology. Several studies have noted an increased incidence of higher pT stage, coagulative tumor necrosis, and sarcomatoid differentiation in the setting of pN1 disease.[12,37] More aggressive biology, even in the presence of metastatic disease, may therefore confer a worse prognosis with rapid systemic progression, obviating the potential benefits of cytoreduction. Moreover, this biology may also explain the observation that nodal stage is independently associated with a worse prognosis, even in the presence of distant metastatic disease.[1]

RENAL CELL CARCINOMA WITH ISOLATED LYMPH NODE METASTASES (pN1 M0 RENAL CELL CARCINOMA)

The natural history of RCC with isolated lymph node metastases not only represents the outcomes of an advanced disease state but, more importantly, provides a unique case study to examine the potential survival benefit of LND. That is, in the nonmetastatic setting, patients with isolated lymph node metastases represent the specific population who may benefit from therapeutic LND, because resection of all sites of nodal metastases should render cure in the setting of otherwise nonmetastatic RCC. To this end, several groups have described the natural history of pN1 M0 RCC.

In the largest single-institution series on the topic of 138 patients with pN1 M0 RCC, the authors reported 5-year metastasis-free survival of only 16%.[40] Moreover, the median time to the development of metastases was only 4.2 months. The authors also identified clinicopathologic features associated with the development of metastases and mortality, which included markers of aggressive disease biology, such as coagulative tumor necrosis, sarcomatoid differentiation, and pT4 stage.[40] In another study of 68 patients with pN1 M0 RCC, only 22.1% were disease free at a median of 43.5 months, and distant recurrence developed within 4 months postoperatively in 51% of patients.[41] Other studies have reported similar oncologic outcomes for pN1 M0 RCC, with 5-year cancer-specific survivals ranging from 22% to 74% and overall survivals from 17% to 53%.[1]

These observations suggest that the overwhelming majority of patients with clinically isolated lymph node metastases harbor occult systemic disease, with rapid progression after surgery. Interestingly, the anatomic basis for the lymphatic drainage of the kidney may explain such behavior. As discussed elsewhere in this article, anatomic mapping studies demonstrate several mechanisms for early hematogeneous dissemination, bypassing the retroperitoneal lymph nodes, including direct communication of efferent lymphatics to the thoracic duct, and direct lymphovenous communications to the renal vein and vena cava.[21]

Still, a small subset of patients demonstrates durable long-term survival.[1] Such patients are more likely to harbor less aggressive tumors. In 1 study, long-term survivors had tumors with lower pT stage and grade, and a lesser incidence of adverse pathologic features.[40] Nonetheless, for the majority of patients, it seems that lymphotropic

RCC tends to reflect an aggressive tumor biology, which portends an ominous prognosis.

MORBIDITY OF LYMPH NODE DISSECTION

In the absence of high-quality data to support a survival benefit, the role of LND is predominantly limited to disease staging. However, if such a role is to be tenable in the management of advanced and/or metastatic RCC, LND cannot be associated with substantial incremental morbidity. To this end, several studies reinforce that, in experienced centers, LND is not associated with increased perioperative morbidity.

In the only randomized data on the topic, EORTC 30881 reported that the performance of LND was not associated with an increase in complications.[9] In that trial, the overall complication rate was 26% for patients undergoing LND compared with 22% for radical nephrectomy alone. Observational studies reinforce these findings. In a secondary analysis of the ASSURE trial, the overall complication rates were 14.2% for LND compared with 13.4% for no LND.[14] In another study, LND was not significantly associated with an increased risk of Clavien grade 3 or higher complications in either M0 or M1 RCC.[42]

SUMMARY

LND does not appear to provide a survival benefit for advanced, nonmetastatic, or metastatic RCC, even in patients at increased risk for lymph node metastases. However, LND serves an important staging role in the management of advanced and metastatic RCC by providing pathologic lymph node stage. LND is not associated with increased perioperative morbidity when performed in experienced centers, which would support a predominantly staging role.

REFERENCES

1. Bhindi B, Wallis CJD, Boorjian SA, et al. The role of lymph node dissection in the management of renal cell carcinoma: a systematic review and meta-analysis. BJU Int 2018;121(5):684–98.
2. Brito J 3rd, Gershman B. The role of lymph node dissection in the contemporary management of renal cell carcinoma: a critical appraisal of the evidence. Urol Oncol 2017;35(11):623–6.
3. Capitanio U, Becker F, Blute ML, et al. Lymph node dissection in renal cell carcinoma. Eur Urol 2011;60(6):1212–20.
4. Barrisford GW, Gershman B, Blute ML Sr. The role of lymphadenectomy in the management of renal cell carcinoma. World J Urol 2014;32(3):643–9.
5. Robson CJ, Churchill BM, Anderson W. The results of radical nephrectomy for renal cell carcinoma. Trans Am Assoc Genitourin Surg 1968;60:122–9.
6. Pantuck AJ, Zisman A, Dorey F, et al. Renal cell carcinoma with retroperitoneal lymph nodes: role of lymph node dissection. J Urol 2003;169(6):2076–83.
7. Schafhauser W, Ebert A, Brod J, et al. Lymph node involvement in renal cell carcinoma and survival chance by systematic lymphadenectomy. Anticancer Res 1999;19(2c):1573–8.
8. Herrlinger A, Schrott KM, Schott G, et al. What are the benefits of extended dissection of the regional renal lymph nodes in the therapy of renal cell carcinoma. J Urol 1991;146(5):1224–7.
9. Blom JH, van Poppel H, Marechal JM, et al. Radical nephrectomy with and without lymph-node dissection: final results of European Organization for Research and Treatment of Cancer (EORTC) randomized phase 3 trial 30881. Eur Urol 2009;55(1):28–34.
10. Feuerstein MA, Kent M, Bazzi WM, et al. Analysis of lymph node dissection in patients with ≥7-cm renal tumors. World J Urol 2014;32(6):1531–6.
11. Feuerstein MA, Kent M, Bernstein M, et al. Lymph node dissection during cytoreductive nephrectomy: a retrospective analysis. Int J Urol 2014;21(9):874–9.
12. Gershman B, Thompson RH, Moreira DM, et al. Lymph node dissection is not associated with improved survival among patients undergoing cytoreductive nephrectomy for metastatic renal cell carcinoma: a propensity score based analysis. J Urol 2017;197(3 Pt 1):574–9.
13. Gershman B, Thompson RH, Moreira DM, et al. Radical nephrectomy with or without lymph node dissection for nonmetastatic renal cell carcinoma: a propensity score-based analysis. Eur Urol 2017;71(4):560–7.
14. Ristau BT, Manola J, Haas NB, et al. Retroperitoneal lymphadenectomy for high risk, nonmetastatic renal cell carcinoma: an analysis of the ASSURE (ECOG-ACRIN 2805) adjuvant trial. J Urol 2018;199(1):53–9.
15. Bekema HJ, MacLennan S, Imamura M, et al. Systematic review of adrenalectomy and lymph node dissection in locally advanced renal cell carcinoma. Eur Urol 2013;64(5):799–810.
16. Motzer RJ, Jonasch E, Agarwal N, et al. Testicular cancer, version 2.2015. J Natl Compr Canc Netw 2015;13(6):772–99.
17. Mohler JL, Armstrong AJ, Bahnson RR, et al. Prostate cancer, version 1.2016. J Natl Compr Canc Netw 2016;14(1):19–30.
18. Campbell S, Uzzo RG, Allaf ME, et al. Renal mass and localized renal cancer: AUA guideline. J Urol 2017;198(3):520–9.
19. Ljungberg B, Bensalah K, Canfield S, et al. EAU guidelines on renal cell carcinoma: 2014 update. Eur Urol 2015;67(5):913–24.

20. Motzer RJ, Jonasch E, Agarwal N, et al. Kidney cancer, version 2.2017, NCCN clinical practice guidelines in oncology. J Natl Compr Canc Netw 2017; 15(6):804–34.

21. Karmali RJ, Suami H, Wood CG, et al. Lymphatic drainage in renal cell carcinoma: back to the basics. BJU Int 2014;114(6):806–17.

22. Kuusk T, De Bruijn R, Brouwer OR, et al. Lymphatic drainage from renal tumors in vivo: a prospective sentinel node study using SPECT/CT imaging. J Urol 2018;199(6):1426–32.

23. Crispen PL, Breau RH, Allmer C, et al. Lymph node dissection at the time of radical nephrectomy for high-risk clear cell renal cell carcinoma: indications and recommendations for surgical templates. Eur Urol 2011;59(1):18–23.

24. Terrone C, Guercio S, De Luca S, et al. The number of lymph nodes examined and staging accuracy in renal cell carcinoma. BJU Int 2003;91(1):37–40.

25. Whitson JM, Harris CR, Reese AC, et al. Lymphadenectomy improves survival of patients with renal cell carcinoma and nodal metastases. J Urol 2011; 185(5):1615–20.

26. Catalano C, Fraioli F, Laghi A, et al. High-resolution multidetector CT in the preoperative evaluation of patients with renal cell carcinoma. AJR Am J Roentgenol 2003;180(5):1271–7.

27. Ergen FB, Hussain HK, Caoili EM, et al. MRI for preoperative staging of renal cell carcinoma using the 1997 TNM classification: comparison with surgical and pathologic staging. AJR Am J Roentgenol 2004;182(1):217–25.

28. Johnson CD, Dunnick NR, Cohan RH, et al. Renal adenocarcinoma: CT staging of 100 tumors. AJR Am J Roentgenol 1987;148(1):59–63.

29. Studer UE, Scherz S, Scheidegger J, et al. Enlargement of regional lymph nodes in renal cell carcinoma is often not due to metastases. J Urol 1990; 144(2 Pt 1):243–5.

30. Gershman B, Takahashi N, Moreira DM, et al. Radiographic size of retroperitoneal lymph nodes predicts pathological nodal involvement for patients with renal cell carcinoma: development of a risk prediction model. BJU Int 2016;118(5):742–9.

31. Blute ML, Leibovich BC, Cheville JC, et al. A protocol for performing extended lymph node dissection using primary tumor pathological features for patients treated with radical nephrectomy for clear cell renal cell carcinoma. J Urol 2004;172(2): 465–9.

32. Babaian KN, Kim DY, Kenney PA, et al. Preoperative predictors of pathological lymph node metastasis in patients with renal cell carcinoma undergoing retroperitoneal lymph node dissection. J Urol 2015; 193(4):1101–7.

33. Capitanio U, Abdollah F, Matloob R, et al. When to perform lymph node dissection in patients with renal cell carcinoma: a novel approach to the preoperative assessment of risk of lymph node invasion at surgery and of lymph node progression during follow-up. BJU Int 2013;112(2):E59–66.

34. Hutterer GC, Patard JJ, Perrotte P, et al. Patients with renal cell carcinoma nodal metastases can be accurately identified: external validation of a new nomogram. Int J Cancer 2007;121(11):2556–61.

35. Lughezzani G, Capitanio U, Jeldres C, et al. Prognostic significance of lymph node invasion in patients with metastatic renal cell carcinoma: a population-based perspective. Cancer 2009; 115(24):5680–7.

36. Trinh QD, Sukumar S, Schmitges J, et al. Effect of nodal metastases on cancer-specific mortality after cytoreductive nephrectomy. Ann Surg Oncol 2013; 20(6):2096–102.

37. Pantuck AJ, Zisman A, Dorey F, et al. Renal cell carcinoma with retroperitoneal lymph nodes. Impact on survival and benefits of immunotherapy. Cancer 2003;97(12):2995–3002.

38. Flanigan RC, Salmon SE, Blumenstein BA, et al. Nephrectomy followed by interferon alfa-2b compared with interferon alfa-2b alone for metastatic renal-cell cancer. N Engl J Med 2001;345(23):1655–9.

39. Mickisch GH, Garin A, van Poppel H, et al. Radical nephrectomy plus interferon-alfa-based immunotherapy compared with interferon alfa alone in metastatic renal-cell carcinoma: a randomised trial. Lancet 2001;358(9286):966–70.

40. Gershman B, Moreira DM, Thompson RH, et al. Renal cell carcinoma with isolated lymph node involvement: long-term natural history and predictors of oncologic outcomes following surgical resection. Eur Urol 2017;72(2):300–6.

41. Delacroix SE Jr, Chapin BF, Chen JJ, et al. Can a durable disease-free survival be achieved with surgical resection in patients with pathological node positive renal cell carcinoma? J Urol 2011;186(4):1236–41.

42. Gershman B, Moreira DM, Thompson RH, et al. Perioperative morbidity of lymph node dissection for renal cell carcinoma: a propensity score-based analysis. Eur Urol 2018;73(3):469–75.

The Evolving Role of Metastasectomy for Patients with Metastatic Renal Cell Carcinoma

Bryan DR Hall, BA, Edwin Jason Abel, MD, FACS*

KEYWORDS

- Metastasectomy • Metastatic renal cell carcinoma • Thermal ablation • Radiation • Immunotherapy
- Targeted therapy • Prognostic factors • Immune checkpoint inhibitors

KEY POINTS

- Surgical metastasectomy may enable periods of systemic treatment-free survival in well-selected patients.
- Ideal patients for metastasectomy are not frail and have a small volume of metastatic disease without aggressive pathologic features.
- The risk of morbidity associated with surgery depends on multiple factors and must be balanced with potential benefits from surgery.
- Prior to metastasectomy, patients should have a multidisciplinary evaluation, including surgeons and medical oncologists, to provide the best shared decision making.

INTRODUCTION

In 1939, Barney and Churchill[1] reported no recurrence of disease for 5 years after a patient was treated with nephrectomy for adenocarcinoma of the kidney and subsequent lobectomy for a 6-cm lung metastasis that was resistant to radiation therapy. Other historical case reports demonstrate that metastasectomy occasionally resulted in long-term survival for patients with metastatic renal cell carcinoma (mRCC), despite having no effective options for systemic therapy in this era.[2] In 1967, Middleton[3] reported 41 patients who had nephrectomy despite known metastatic disease treated from 1932 to 1965 at New York Hospital. The reported overall survival was significantly better for patients with solitary metastasis, most of whom were treated with metastasectomy. Long-term survivors included a patient, who was alive without recurrence, 31 years after the initial nephrectomy and 14 years after excision of a brain metastasis.

The rare opportunity to provide long-term, disease-free survival for a subset of patients with solitary metastasis provided a rationale for metastasectomy before active systemic treatments became available. More recently, patients with oligometastatic renal cell carcinoma (RCC) have been treated with metastasectomy after partial responses to cytokine therapy[4] or targeted therapies.[5] However, the benefit of surgery as a local treatment for RCC metastases is difficult to measure accurately because benefits are confined to a small fraction of patients and no large randomized clinical trials having investigated metastasectomy for typical mRCC patients. Furthermore, surgeons intentionally choose lower-risk patients with slow-growing metastases

Funding: None.
Department of Urology, University of Wisconsin School of Medicine and Public Health, 1685 Highland Avenue, Madison, WI 53705, USA
* Corresponding author.
E-mail address: abel@urology.wisc.edu

Urol Clin N Am 47 (2020) 379–388
https://doi.org/10.1016/j.ucl.2020.04.012
0094-0143/20/Published by Elsevier Inc.

for metastasectomy, creating an observation bias when comparing outcomes.

Over the past 2 decades, systemic treatments that target angiogenesis or cell growth pathways have demonstrated prolonged survival compared to patients treated with interferon-α in large randomized clinical trials.[6,7] Although better systemic treatments for mRCC became increasingly available, the utilization of metastasectomy continued to increase from 2006 to 2013.[8] More recently, single-agent[9] or combination therapies[10] that target immunologic checkpoints have emerged as first-line systemic therapies. In 2019, new combination treatments using both targeted therapies and immune checkpoint inhibitors gained approval for mRCC treatment after demonstrating improved survival in clinical trials.[11,12] Metastasectomy may be less utilized with complete responses, which are more common with newer therapies (9% complete response rate for patients treated with nivolimab plus ipilimumab).[10] Metastasectomy, however, is likely to continue to play a role in the multidisciplinary treatment of mRCC until systemic therapies produce complete and durable responses. The purpose of this review is to examine the currently available data for metastasectomy in mRCC patients, including site-specific data and strategies for patient selection.

UTILIZATION OF METASTASECTOMY FOR METASTATIC RENAL CELL CARCINOMA

Studies that estimate how often mRCC patients are treated with metastasectomy were uncommon before the development of large cancer registries. Furthermore, improvements in imaging technology during the past few decades have resulted in earlier detection of smaller asymptomatic metastases, which also may have an impact on the utilization of metastasectomy,[13] which also may vary significantly among institutions. For example, in a single-institution series of 887 mRCC patients from 1976 to 2006, 48% of patients had surgical resection of metastases.[14] Sun and colleagues[8] evaluated population-level data from the National Cancer Database and found 1976/6994 (28%) patients with mRCC were treated with metastasectomy from 2006 to 2013 and that utilization increased from 24.9% in 2006 to 31.4% in 2013.[8] Increased utilization of metastasectomy in recent years has not been limited to kidney cancer. Bartlett and colleagues[15] found that metastasectomy increased from 2000 to 2011 across many cancer types, including colorectal, lung, breast, and melanoma. Increase in utilization was greatest in colorectal cancer, which had the most efficacious systemic therapy during the study period.[15]

EVIDENCE FOR METASTASECTOMY IN METASTATIC RENAL CELL CARCINOMA

Multiple reviews and meta-analyses are available to systematically evaluate the evidence for surgery in the treatment of RCC metastases.[16–19] In 2018, Ouzaid and colleagues[16] systematically reviewed the literature and found that median overall survival for patients treated with metastasectomy (36–142 months) was higher compared with patients treated without metastasectomy (8–27 months). Investigating the concept of complete versus incomplete surgical metastasectomy also provides evidence for the possible impact of surgical treatments. Alt and colleagues[14] evaluated 887 patients with multiple RCC metastases from 1976 to 2006, including 125 who had complete surgical metastasectomy. The median cancer-specific and overall survival rates for patients who underwent complete metastasectomy were 4.8 years and 4.0 years, respectively, compared with 1.3 years and 1.3 years, for patients who did not undergo complete metastasectomy. There was a survival benefit provided by complete metastasectomy compared with incomplete metastasectomy when patients had 2 or more metastases.[14] Patients treated surgically, however, had significant differences in disease burden and performance status compared with the nonsurgically treated patients.[14] In a subsequent article from the same institution, evaluating 586 patients with first occurrence of metastases between 2006 and 2017, 158 patients were treated with complete metastasectomy.[20] After adjusting for age, sex, timing, number, and location of metastases, the investigators found that complete metastasectomy was associated with reduced likelihood of death from RCC (hazard ratio 0.47; 95% CI, 0.34–0.65; $P<.001$).[20] Collectively, these data suggest improved survival for patients treated with complete metastasectomy was better than incomplete metastasectomy or no local treatment, although this concept should be investigated in multi-institutional cohorts.

PATIENT SELECTION

Patient selection is critical to achieve optimal outcomes, and metastasectomy for mRCC is one of the best examples of this surgical maxim. Factors associated with improved outcomes after metastasectomy include (1) smaller volume of metastatic disease, (2) slower disease progression, and (3) lack of competing caused for mortality. Prior to metastasectomy, patients should consult with a multidisciplinary team and discuss expectations for outcomes based on individual considerations (**Fig. 1**).

Overall patient health is important to consider prior to surgery (see **Fig. 1**A). Patients with limited life expectancy because of comorbidities are less likely to benefit from surgery. Although metastasectomy is more likely to be utilized in younger patients,[8] actual patient age may be less important than physiologic age, which is associated with treatment outcomes in older patients with cancer.[21] Performance status is a critical factor associated with survival in mRCC[22] and surgeons should consider patients with better performance status for metastasectomy. It is important, however, to consider how surgery may affect short-term and long-term performance status. Occasionally, performance status may improve for patients with symptomatic metastasis, such as patients with pathologic bone fractures or gross hematuria. Furthermore, because major adverse events of systemic therapies also affect performance status, surgery may improve performance status by delaying systemic therapy and potential adverse events in some patients.

Cancer-specific survival in mRCC patients varies significantly, with many known tumor specific prognostic factors (see **Fig. 1**B). In general, patients with solitary or low-volume metastatic disease and fewer sites of metastasis have longer expected survival.[23] In addition, patients with initially localized tumors and a longer time from nephrectomy to metastatic diagnosis are more likely to survive longer compared with patients with synchronous metastatic disease.[24] Several validated risk assessment tools estimate overall survival in mRCC[24,25] and may be useful for patients considering metastasectomy.[26] Observed radiographic growth of metastatic tumors also is important as a prognostic factor for survival,[27] and some patients with slow-growing metastases may be observed safely without systemic treatment.[28] Tumor growth despite systemic treatment is associated with poor survival[29] and these patients are unlikely to benefit from aggressive surgery. Rapid progression also is associated with aggressive pathologic features, such as sarcomatoid de-differentiation, and upfront cytoreductive surgery, generally is not recommended.[30] Similarly, Thomas and colleagues[31] found no benefit for metastasectomy after nephrectomy in

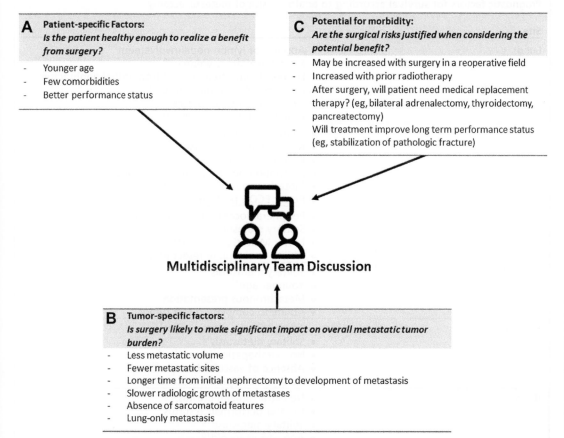

A Patient-specific Factors:
Is the patient healthy enough to realize a benefit from surgery?

- Younger age
- Few comorbidities
- Better performance status

C Potential for morbidity:
Are the surgical risks justified when considering the potential benefit?

- May be increased with surgery in a reoperative field
- Increased with prior radiotherapy
- After surgery, will patient need medical replacement therapy? (eg, bilateral adrenalectomy, thyroidectomy, pancreatectomy)
- Will treatment improve long term performance status (eg, stabilization of pathologic fracture)

Multidisciplinary Team Discussion

B Tumor-specific factors:
Is surgery likely to make significant impact on overall metastatic tumor burden?

- Less metastatic volume
- Fewer metastatic sites
- Longer time from initial nephrectomy to development of metastasis
- Slower radiologic growth of metastases
- Absence of sarcomatoid features
- Lung-only metastasis

Fig. 1. Prior to metastasectomy, mRCC patients should be counseled by a multidisciplinary team. Using a shared decision-making approach, the treatment team should discuss individual (*A*) patient-specific factors, (*B*) tumor-specific factors, and (*C*) potential for morbidity with surgery or systemic agents.

a matched-pair analysis of mRCC patients with sarcomatoid de-differentiation.

In addition to the patient-specific and tumor-specific factors, shared decision making before metastasectomy should consider the possible short-term and long-term morbidity associated with surgical treatment (see **Fig. 1**C). Morbidity varies with the type of procedure, approach, and anatomic location but may be comparable to other surgeries for primary tumors at those anatomic locations.[16] Surgery may be more complex if scarring is present from prior surgery or tissues are poor quality because of prior radiation therapy. In addition, treatment with targeted therapies for mRCC are associated with wound-healing complications[32] and surgery requires interruption of certain systemic treatments. Other considerations to consider may be the need for medical replacement of hormones after adrenalectomy, thyroidectomy, or pancreatectomy. Informed consent should include a balanced discussion of the risks of surgical as well as the systemic therapies. Given the multiple unique medical and surgical factors to consider before metastasectomy, discussion with a multidisciplinary team of surgeons and medical oncologists is recommended.

INDIVIDUAL METASTATIC SITES

Certain anatomic sites and prognostic factors may be associated with better outcomes in with mRCC metastasectomy sites (**Table 1**). Some anatomic sites are more surgically more accessible, and procedures may be less morbid. For example, patients treated with a minimally invasive wedge resection of a small lung metastasis are exposed to less risk of surgical morbidity compared with an open resection of large liver metastases. More importantly, some metastatic sites are associated with slower disease progression. For example, pancreatic RCC metastatic tumors frequently are

Table 1 Prognostic factors for survival according to anatomic site of metastasectomy	
Site	
Lung	• Absence of lymph node involvement[79] • Forced expiratory volume[79] • Longer disease-free interval from initial nephrectomy[79] • Fewer number of metastases[79] • Smaller size of metastases[17] • Unilateral lung involvement[17]
Liver	• Solitary metastasis[17] • No extrahepatic disease[17] • Low tumor grade[17] • No lymph node metastasis at initial diagnosis[42] • Metachronous presentation[42] • Better ECOG performance status[42]
Bone	• Peripheral location of metastases[18] • Solitary metastases[17] • Lower MSKCC risk score[46] • Ability to complete resect tumor[46]
Thyroid	• Solitary metastasis[17] • Younger age[17] • Metachronous presentation • Ability to complete resect tumor
Pancreas	• Asymptomatic presentation[17] • Solitary metastasis[17] • No extrahepatic disease[17] • Absence of vascular invasion[80] • Ability to complete resect tumor
Brain	• No extracranial metastasis[17] • Greater performance status[17] • Solitary metastasis[18] • Age $\leq$65 years old[18] • Control of primary tumor[18]

Data from Refs.[17,18,42,46,79,80]

observed to be slow growing and patients with pancreatic metastasis may have longer survival compared with those with metastasis at other sites.[33] Clinical observations from multiple centers have confirmed these observations and demonstrated that metastasectomy is a feasible treatment in patients with pancreatic RCC metastases.[34] Recently, basic science evidence has emerged that may begin to explain the slower natural history of pancreatic metastasis. In 2018, Turajlic and colleagues[35] observed that pancreatic metastasis had the longest time to presentation of all RCC metastases, which was associated with significantly less chromosomal instability and few additional driver mutations despite longer time to clinical detection.

Pulmonary Metastasectomy

The lungs are the most common site of metastasis for RCC,[36] and pulmonary resections are the most common type of metastasectomy described for mRCC. When investigating survival benefit among anatomic sites of RCC metastasis, a systematic review suggested that pulmonary metastasectomy has the strongest association with a survival benefit.[16] In a meta-analysis of studies evaluating pulmonary metastasectomy for mRCC, poor prognostic factors for survival after pulmonary metastasectomy included multiple pulmonary metastases, incomplete resection, larger size of pulmonary metastasis, lymphatic invasion, and synchronous presentation of metastasis.[19]

Multiple open and video-assisted thoracoscopic surgery (VATS) surgical approaches are used routinely for pulmonary metastasectomy. Expert consensus from the Society of Thoracic Surgeons (STS) recommends using minimally invasive techniques when appropriate for metastasectomy.[37] In general, VATS is used for small solitary unilateral lesions whereas open thoracotomy is used when the lesions are larger and bilateral. In a National Cancer Database population-based cohort, mRCC patients with lung metastasis had significantly better survival at 1 year, 2 years, and 3 years if they were treated with metastasectomy (78%, 59%, and 47%, respectively) versus nonsurgical management (65%, 45%, and 34%).[8] In addition to lung parenchymal metastases, metastatic tumor may be present in the mediastinal lymph nodes or based in the pleura.[38] As such, the STS recommends regional lymph node sampling when clinically suspicious.[37] Long-term survival after mediastinal metastasectomy has been reported[39] but fewer data are available compared with lung parenchymal metastases.

Hepatic Metastasectomy

Liver metastasis is present in approximately 20% of mRCC patients.[36] Historically, liver resection of mRCC lesions was uncommon due to the higher morbidity associated with hepatic surgery.[40] Overall, hepatic metastasis appears associated with poor oncologic outcomes compared with RCC metastasis at other sites.[41] When considering hepatic resection for mRCC, improved overall survival is associated with complete resection, metachronous presentation of metastases, lower primary tumor grade, better Eastern Cooperative Oncology Group (ECOG) status, and lack of extrahepatic metastatic sites.[16] Staehler and colleagues[42] identified 88 patients with liver metastases between 1995 and 2006. A total of 68 patients were treated with liver resection and 20 were managed nonsurgically, serving as a control cohort. The investigators found that metachronous liver metastases treated surgically were associated with significantly better survival compared with the control group, 155 versus 29 months, respectively.[42] The investigators found that hepatic metastasectomy was associated with 5-year survival of 62% but suggest that no benefit is present if metastases are synchronous.[42] In a multi-institutional study of 43 hepatic metastasectomy patients from 1994 to 2011, Hatzaras and colleagues[40] reported a 3-year overall survival rate of 62% and a median length of recurrence-free survival of 15.5 months. No differences in positive margin rates, recurrence, or survival were identified for parenchymal sparing versus anatomic liver resection techniques.[43] Because of the higher risk of morbidity with hepatic surgery, nonsurgical local treatments for liver metastases using radiation or thermal ablation also are common.[18,44]

Bone Metastasectomy

Bone metastases are another common site of RCC metastasis, identified in approximately 30% of mRCC patients,[36] most commonly in the spinal column.[45] One study investigating prognostic factors for mRCC patients with bone metastases found that Memorial Sloan Kettering Cancer Center (MSKCC) risk score, increased number of bone metastases, and radical resection were important prognostic factors for survival.[46] The investigators concluded that surgery with the intention of gaining local tumor control should be considered if a patient presents with solitary bone lesions without concomitant metastases at the initial diagnosis, which may be associated with better overall survival.[46]

When evaluating overall survival, local therapy combined with targeted therapy had superior overall survival benefit compared with local therapy or targeted therapy alone.[47] Median overall survival rate of patients with bone metastases resection (n = 33) was 39.1 months and was significantly longer than those of the patients with resection of any other site (n = 22) and patients without metastasis (n = 59), which were 8.3 months and 7.6 months, respectively.[47] Comparing metastasectomy with no metastasectomy, there was a significant difference between the median overall survival of 17.79 versus 8.71 months.[48] For patients who present with bone metastases who are not surgical candidates, radiation therapy and thermal ablation are local therapy options. A recent systematic review reviewed stereotactic body radiotherapy (SBRT) for mRCC spinal metastases and concluded that there was pain improved in 41% to 95% of patients and that local control rates after stereotactic radiation ranged from 71.2% to 85.7% at 1 year.[49] Toxicity rates ranged from 23% to 38.5%, and there was an increased risk of vertebral compression fracture after treatment.

Pancreatic Metastasectomy

As discussed previously, pancreatic metastases from RCC frequently have been observed to be less aggressive,[33] but morbidity from pancreatic surgery also may be more significant than other anatomic sites. In a series of 97 patients treated with 98 pancreatic metastasectomies from July 1988 through March 2016 for metastatic disease, postoperative complications were reported in 56% patients and perioperative deaths occurred in 3% of patients.[50] Median follow-up was 2.0 years and median survival was 3.2 years. Older patients, non-RCC histology, vascular invasion, and positive resection margins were independently associated with an increased risk of mortality.[50]

A recent systematic review of resection of pancreatic metastasis included 414 pancreatic metastasectomies (techniques included pancreatoduodenectomy 38%, total pancreatectomy 11%, distal pancreatectomy 43%, and enucleation 7%). Overall morbidity and mortality rates were 48.3% and 1.4%, respectively.[51] The investigators concluded that pancreatic metastasectomy was a safe option at experienced centers. Lee and colleagues[50] demonstrated a median survival for 56 patients with resected RCC pancreatic metastases of 4.8 years, which is similar to that in other studies, with 5-year overall survival rates of 48% to 72%.[50–52]

Thyroid Metastasectomy

Although head and neck metastases from mRCC are less common overall, thyroid metastases are well described.[53] In the thyroid gland, metastases usually are single (77%) and unilateral (71%).[53,54] A survival advantage for thyroidectomy has been suggested in isolated singular and multiple metastases.[14,55] The current guidelines of the European Association of Urology recommend metastasectomy in cases of a resectable lesion regardless of the site, whether synchronous or metachronous.[53] No significant survival difference has been shown between total thyroidectomy and subtotal thyroidectomy.[53,56,57] Recurrence in those managed with partial thyroidectomy may be high (20%), which may be related to the presence of positive margins at initial surgery or multifocal disease.[53] Outcomes with thyroid metastases generally are favorable[57,58] with overall 5-year and 10-year survival rates for patients with isolated metachronous thyroid metastasis who underwent metastasectomy being 51.4% and 25.7%, respectively.[56]

Adrenal Gland Metastasectomy

Although the classic description of radical nephrectomy for RCC included ipsilateral adrenalectomy,[59] Weight and colleagues[60] found that ipsilateral adrenalectomy did not lower the risk of subsequent metastasis or improve survival in patients with localized RCC. The 10-year risk for the development of an ipsilateral or contralateral asynchronous adrenal metastasis was equivocal for patients treated with adrenalectomy at the time of nephrectomy.[60] For patients who present with metachronous metastatic tumors in the adrenal gland, minimally invasive surgical techniques may be used,[61] even for adrenalectomy after previous ipsilateral nephrectomy.[62] An open approach may be preferred when periadrenal fat invasion is suspected, when tumor thrombus is present, or for tumors greater than 10 cm.[63] In a study of 1179 patients where 45 had adrenal metastasis, patients with isolated adrenal metastasis survived significantly longer than those with multiple metastasis.[64] Surgical curative outcomes were demonstrated in 10 cases without relapse at a mean follow-up of 82.9 months.[64]

Brain Metastasectomy

RCC metastasis to the brain has a reported incidence of 2% to 17%[65] and multiple reports of curative treatment with complete resection have been published. Historically, brain metastases have been thought to be associated with poor outcomes, although recent contradictory evidence has suggested that patients with brain metastases may have similar outcomes to other metastatic sites with aggressive treatment.[66] Time to development of metastasis appears to be an important prognostic factor, with brain metastases presenting more than 10 years after the initial RCC diagnosis associated with favorable outcomes.[67] Multiple studies have identified favorable outcomes for some patients with solitary RCC brain metastases after local treatment.[8,66]

MORBIDITY OF TREATMENTS FOR METASTATIC RENAL CELL CARCINOMA

Although systemic therapies have improved survival for mRCC patients greatly, there are significant risks of severe adverse events.[68] Prior to treatment, mRCC patients should discuss the likelihood of adverse events and may consider potential benefits of local treatments. Although many studies have demonstrated low morbidity with surgical metastasectomy,[16] there are conflicting data from population-based studies. Using the National Inpatient Sample database between 2000 and 2011, Meyer and colleagues[69] identified 45,279 patients with mRCC, including 1102 treated with metastasectomy. Overall complications and major complications (Clavien-Dindo III-IV) were identified in 46% and 25%, respectively, of patients, with in-hospital mortality of 2.4%. In a similar study of mRCC treated with metastasectomy from the National Inpatient Sample database between 2006 and 2015, overall complications and in-hospital mortality were 55% and 4.6%, respectively.[70] Potential explanations for the discrepancy in morbidity rates between studies may include the difficulty of accurate recording of complications for rare procedures. Alternatively, higher-volume centers may be more likely to publish data for metastasectomy,[16] which may be skewed because of better outcomes demonstrated at centers with higher volume of mRCC patients.[71] Age, comorbidities, and hepatic surgery are associated with higher risk of major complications.[69]

RADIATION OR PERCUTANEOUS THERMAL ABLATION FOR LOCAL METASTATIC RENAL CELL CARCINOMA TREATMENT

Alternatives to surgical metastasectomy include radiation and thermal ablation. No high-quality data are available to compare outcomes between surgery and other local treatments directly, but there may be potential advantages for some patients and anatomic locations. For example, radiation and thermal ablation may not require general anesthesia and have shorter recovery. Accordingly, the potential benefits of nonsurgical treatments must be balanced with the expected durability of results and goals of therapy in order to select patients appropriately.

Historically, RCC was considered a radioresistant tumor but more recent studies have demonstrated success with SBRT.[72] A recent meta-analysis included 28 studies with 1602 patients and 3892 lesions (1159 extracranial/2733 intracranial).[72] Local control rates were approximately 90% at 1 year and clavien grade III-IV toxicities were identified in approximately 1% of patients. Especially in more frail patients with bone metastases, SBRT may be an effective treatment to decrease pain.[73] Thermal ablation also has been described as a local treatment of mRCC using radiofrequency ablation, cryoablation, or microwave ablation. Percutaneous approaches generally are used with ultrasound or computerized tomography for guidance.

A study by Welch and colleagues[74] evaluated percutaneous image-guided ablations for 61 mRCC patients treated with ablation procedures and found local recurrence-free and overall survival rates at 3 years after ablation were 83% and 76%, respectively. Similarly, Maciolek and colleagues[75] evaluated 18 patients treated with percutaneous microwave ablation for 33 mRCC sites between 2011 and 2016. The ablation locations included the retroperitoneum, contralateral kidney, liver, lung, and adrenal gland. Technical success was achieved for all mRCC tumors and local control was achieved for 28/30 (93%) mRCC tumors, with a median follow-up of 1.6 years. One Clavien grade III complication was identified and the estimated 5-year overall survival was 75%.

COST OF LOCAL VERSUS SYSTEMIC THERAPIES

In addition to delaying adverse events from systemic therapy, it has been suggested that local treatment of mRCC also may be cost effective by delaying or possibly avoiding systemic therapies in a subset of patients.[17] With newer therapies and differences in health care systems direct comparisons are difficult. The annual cost of targeted drug therapies, however, is estimated at $125,000 to $200,000.[76] Furthermore, cost of systemic treatment may increase for additional lines of therapy. In a study that evaluated cost of switching among different treatment mRCC regimens used for first-line, second-line, and third-line mRCC treatments in 767 patients, the investigators found that total costs per patient during the first year increased from \$111,680 for no drug switches; \$149,994 for 1 switch; and \$196,706 for 2 or more switches.[76] Given that the cost of metastasectomy[77] or thermal ablation[78] is significantly less than systemic therapies in many health care systems, local treatment potentially may decrease overall treatment costs if systemic therapies can be delayed or avoided in some patients.

SUMMARY

The primary rationale for local treatment of mRCC is that metastasectomy may provide systemic treatment-free survival for a subset of patients. Patient selection is critical for optimal outcomes and metastasectomy is less likely to benefit patients who are frail or have aggressive tumor behavior. Utilization of surgical metastasectomy continues to increase despite improved mRCC systemic therapies over the past 2 decades. Future studies will evaluate the optimal role of metastasectomy with newer therapies. Patients considering metastasectomy should receive multidisciplinary evaluation to improved shared decision making.

CONFLICTS OF INTEREST

The authors have nothing to disclose.

REFERENCES

1. Barney JD, Churchill EJ. Adenocarcinoma of the kidney with metastasis to the lung - Cured by nephrectomy and lobectomy. J Urol 1939;42(3):269–76.
2. Clark WS, Mccort JJ, Mallory TB, et al. Metastatic renal adenocarcinoma. N Engl J Med 1948; 238(26):915–8.
3. Middleton RG. Surgery for metastatic renal cell carcinoma. J Urol 1967;97(6):973–7.
4. Daliani DD, Tannir NM, Papandreou CN, et al. Prospective assessment of systemic therapy followed by surgical removal of metastases in selected patients with renal cell carcinoma. BJU Int 2009; 104(4):456–60.
5. Karam JA, Rini BI, Varella L, et al. Metastasectomy after targeted therapy in patients with advanced renal cell carcinoma. J Urol 2011;185(2):439–44.
6. Escudier B, Eisen T, Stadler WM, et al. Sorafenib in advanced clear-cell renal-cell carcinoma. N Engl J Med 2007;356(2):125–34.
7. Motzer RJ, Hutson TE, Tomczak P, et al. Sunitinib versus interferon alfa in metastatic renal-cell carcinoma. N Engl J Med 2007;356(2):115–24.
8. Sun M, Meyer CP, Karam JA, et al. Predictors, utilization patterns, and overall survival of patients undergoing metastasectomy for metastatic renal cell carcinoma in the era of targeted therapy. Eur J Surg Oncol 2018;44(9):1439–45.

9. Motzer RJ, Escudier B, McDermott DF, et al. Nivolumab versus everolimus in advanced renal-cell carcinoma. N Engl J Med 2015;373(19):1803–13.
10. Motzer RJ, Tannir NM, McDermott DF, et al. Nivolumab plus ipilimumab versus sunitinib in advanced renal-cell carcinoma. N Engl J Med 2018;378(14): 1277–90.
11. Motzer RJ, Penkov K, Haanen J, et al. Avelumab plus axitinib versus sunitinib for advanced renal-cell carcinoma. N Engl J Med 2019;380(12): 1103–15.
12. Rini BI, Plimack ER, Stus V, et al. Pembrolizumab plus axitinib versus sunitinib for advanced renal-cell carcinoma. N Engl J Med 2019;380(12): 1116–27.
13. Dabestani S, Beisland C, Stewart GD, et al. Long-term outcomes of follow-up for initially localised clear cell renal cell carcinoma: RECUR database analysis. Eur Urol Focus 2019;5(5):857–66.
14. Alt AL, Boorjian SA, Lohse CM, et al. Survival after complete surgical resection of multiple metastases from renal cell carcinoma. Cancer 2011;117(13): 2873–82.
15. Bartlett EK, Simmons KD, Wachtel H, et al. The rise in metastasectomy across cancer types over the past decade. Cancer 2015;121(5):747–57.
16. Ouzaid I, Capitanio U, Staehler M, et al. Surgical metastasectomy in renal cell carcinoma: a systematic review. Eur Urol Oncol 2019;2(2):141–9.
17. Psutka SP, Master VA. Role of metastasis-directed treatment in kidney cancer. Cancer 2018;124(18): 3641–55.
18. Dabestani S, Marconi L, Hofmann F, et al. Local treatments for metastases of renal cell carcinoma: a systematic review. Lancet Oncol 2014;15(12): e549–61.
19. Zhao Y, Li J, Li C, et al. Prognostic factors for overall survival after lung metastasectomy in renal cell cancer patients: A systematic review and meta-analysis. Int J Surg 2017;41:70–7.
20. Lyon TD, Thompson RH, Shah PH, et al. Complete surgical metastasectomy of renal cell carcinoma in the post-cytokine era. J Urol 2020 Feb;203(2): 275–82.
21. Wildiers H, Heeren P, Puts M, et al. International Society of Geriatric Oncology consensus on geriatric assessment in older patients with cancer. J Clin Oncol 2014;32(24):2595–603.
22. Xu Y, Zhang Y, Wang X, et al. Prognostic value of performance status in metastatic renal cell carcinoma patients receiving tyrosine kinase inhibitors: a systematic review and meta-analysis. BMC Cancer 2019;19(1):168.
23. Han KR, Pantuck AJ, Bui MH, et al. Number of metastatic sites rather than location dictates overall survival of patients with node-negative metastatic renal cell carcinoma. Urology 2003;61(2):314–9.

24. Motzer RJ, Mazumdar M, Bacik J, et al. Survival and prognostic stratification of 670 patients with advanced renal cell carcinoma. J Clin Oncol 1999; 17(8):2530–40.

25. Heng DY, Xie W, Regan MM, et al. Prognostic factors for overall survival in patients with metastatic renal cell carcinoma treated with vascular endothelial growth factor-targeted agents: results from a large, multicenter study. J Clin Oncol 2009;27(34): 5794–9.

26. Eggener SE, Yossepowitch O, Kundu S, et al. Risk score and metastasectomy independently impact prognosis of patients with recurrent renal cell carcinoma. J Urol 2008;180(3):873–8 [discussion: 878].

27. Stein WD, Huang H, Menefee M, et al. Other paradigms: growth rate constants and tumor burden determined using computed tomography data correlate strongly with the overall survival of patients with renal cell carcinoma. Cancer J 2009;15(5): 441–7.

28. Rini BI, Dorff TB, Elson P, et al. Active surveillance in metastatic renal-cell carcinoma: a prospective, phase 2 trial. Lancet Oncol 2016;17(9):1317–24.

29. Heng DY, Mackenzie MJ, Vaishampayan UN, et al. Primary anti-vascular endothelial growth factor (VEGF)-refractory metastatic renal cell carcinoma: clinical characteristics, risk factors, and subsequent therapy. Ann Oncol 2012;23(6):1549–55.

30. Shapiro DD, Abel EJ. Patient selection for cytoreductive nephrectomy in combination with targeted therapies or immune checkpoint inhibitors. Curr Opin Urol 2019;29(5):513–20.

31. Thomas AZ, Adibi M, Slack RS, et al. The role of metastasectomy in patients with renal cell carcinoma with sarcomatoid dedifferentiation: a matched controlled analysis. J Urol 2016;196(3):678–84.

32. Chapin BF, Delacroix SE Jr, Culp SH, et al. Safety of presurgical targeted therapy in the setting of metastatic renal cell carcinoma. Eur Urol 2011;60(5): 964–71.

33. Kalra S, Atkinson BJ, Matrana MR, et al. Prognosis of patients with metastatic renal cell carcinoma and pancreatic metastases. BJU Int 2016;117(5):761–5.

34. Grassi P, Doucet L, Giglione P, et al. Clinical impact of pancreatic metastases from renal cell carcinoma: a multicenter retrospective analysis. PLoS One 2016;11(4):e0151662.

35. Turajlic S, Xu H, Litchfield K, et al. Tracking cancer evolution reveals constrained routes to metastases: TRACERx renal. Cell 2018;173(3):581–594 e512.

36. Bianchi M, Sun M, Jeldres C, et al. Distribution of metastatic sites in renal cell carcinoma: a population-based analysis. Ann Oncol 2012;23(4): 973–80.

37. Handy JR, Bremner RM, Crocenzi TS, et al. Expert consensus document on pulmonary metastasectomy. Ann Thorac Surg 2019;107(2):631–49.

38. Kutty K, Varkey B. Incidence and distribution of intrathoracic metastases from renal cell carcinoma. Arch Intern Med 1984;144(2):273–6.

39. Takanami I, Naruke M, Kodaira S. Long-term survival after resection of a mediastinal metastasis from a renal cell carcinoma. J Thorac Cardiovasc Surg 1998;115(5):1218–9.

40. Hatzaras I, Gleisner AL, Pulitano C, et al. A multi-institution analysis of outcomes of liver-directed surgery for metastatic renal cell cancer. HPB (Oxford) 2012;14(8):532–8.

41. McKay RR, Kroeger N, Xie W, et al. Impact of bone and liver metastases on patients with renal cell carcinoma treated with targeted therapy. Eur Urol 2014; 65(3):577–84.

42. Staehler MD, Kruse J, Haseke N, et al. Liver resection for metastatic disease prolongs survival in renal cell carcinoma: 12-year results from a retrospective comparative analysis. World J Urol 2010;28(4): 543–7.

43. Moris D, Ronnekleiv-Kelly S, Rahnemai-Azar AA, et al. Parenchymal-sparing versus anatomic liver resection for colorectal liver metastases: a systematic review. J Gastrointest Surg 2017;21(6): 1076–85.

44. Goering JD, Mahvi DM, Niederhuber JE, et al. Cryoablation and liver resection for noncolorectal liver metastases. Am J Surg 2002;183(4):384–9.

45. Shvarts O, Lam JS, Kim HL, et al. Eastern Cooperative Oncology Group performance status predicts bone metastasis in patients presenting with renal cell carcinoma: implication for preoperative bone scans. J Urol 2004;172(3):867–70.

46. Ruatta F, Derosa L, Escudier B, et al. Prognosis of renal cell carcinoma with bone metastases: Experience from a large cancer centre. Eur J Cancer 2019;107:79–85.

47. Du Y, Pahernik S, Hadaschik B, et al. Survival and prognostic factors of patients with renal cell cancer with bone metastasis in the era of targeted therapy: A single-institution analysis. Urol Oncol 2016;34(10): 433.e1-8.

48. Kim SH, Park WS, Park B, et al. A retrospective analysis of the impact of metastasectomy on prognostic survival according to metastatic organs in patients with metastatic renal cell carcinoma. Front Oncol 2019;9:413.

49. Smith BW, Joseph JR, Saadeh YS, et al. Radiosurgery for treatment of renal cell metastases to spine: a systematic review of the literature. World Neurosurg 2018;109:e502–9.

50. Lee SR, Gemenetzis G, Cooper M, et al. Long-term outcomes of 98 surgically resected metastatic tumors in the pancreas. Ann Surg Oncol 2017;24(3): 801–7.

51. Huang Q, Zhou H, Liu C, et al. Surgical resection for metastatic tumors in the pancreas: a single-center

experience and systematic review. Ann Surg Oncol 2019;26(6):1649–56.

52. Reddy S, Wolfgang CL. The role of surgery in the management of isolated metastases to the pancreas. Lancet Oncol 2009;10(3):287–93.

53. Montero PH, Ibrahimpasic T, Nixon IJ, et al. Thyroid metastasectomy. J Surg Oncol 2014;109(1):36–41.

54. Sindoni A, Rizzo M, Tuccari G, et al. Thyroid metastases from renal cell carcinoma: review of the literature. ScientificWorldJournal 2010;10:590–602.

55. Kavolius JP, Mastorakos DP, Pavlovich C, et al. Resection of metastatic renal cell carcinoma. J Clin Oncol 1998;16(6):2261–6.

56. Heffess CS, Wenig BM, Thompson LD. Metastatic renal cell carcinoma to the thyroid gland: a clinicopathologic study of 36 cases. Cancer 2002;95(9):1869–78.

57. Wood K, Vini L, Harmer C. Metastases to the thyroid gland: the Royal Marsden experience. Eur J Surg Oncol 2004;30(6):583–8.

58. Nakhjavani MK, Gharib H, Goellner JR, et al. Metastasis to the thyroid gland. A report of 43 cases. Cancer 1997;79(3):574–8.

59. Robson CJ, Churchill BM, Anderson W. The results of radical nephrectomy for renal cell carcinoma. J Urol 1969;101(3):297–301.

60. Weight CJ, Kim SP, Lohse CM, et al. Routine adrenalectomy in patients with locally advanced renal cell cancer does not offer oncologic benefit and places a significant portion of patients at risk for an asynchronous metastasis in a solitary adrenal gland. Eur Urol 2011;60(3):458–64.

61. Carr AA, Wang TS. Minimally invasive adrenalectomy. Surg Oncol Clin N Am 2016;25(1):139–52.

62. Abel EJ, Karam JA, Carrasco A, et al. Laparoscopic adrenalectomy for metachronous metastases after ipsilateral nephrectomy for renal-cell carcinoma. J Endourol 2011;25(8):1323–7.

63. Taffurelli G, Ricci C, Casadei R, et al. Open adrenalectomy in the era of laparoscopic surgery: a review. Updates Surg 2017;69(2):135–43.

64. Antonelli A, Cozzoli A, Simeone C, et al. Surgical treatment of adrenal metastasis from renal cell carcinoma: a single-centre experience of 45 patients. BJU Int 2006;97(3):505–8.

65. Shuch B, La Rochelle JC, Klatte T, et al. Brain metastasis from renal cell carcinoma: presentation, recurrence, and survival. Cancer 2008;113(7):1641–8.

66. Bowman IA, Bent A, Le T, et al. Improved survival outcomes for kidney cancer patients with brain metastases. Clin Genitourin Cancer 2019;17(2):e263–72.

67. Fukushima Y, Yoshikawa G, Takasago M, et al. Extremely delayed multiple brain metastases from renal cell carcinoma: remission achieved with total surgical removal: case report and literature review. World Neurosurg 2016;92:583.e3-7.

68. Pal S, Gong J, Mhatre SK, et al. Real-world treatment patterns and adverse events in metastatic renal cell carcinoma from a large US claims database. BMC Cancer 2019;19(1):548.

69. Meyer CP, Sun M, Karam JA, et al. Complications after metastasectomy for renal cell carcinoma-a population-based assessment. Eur Urol 2017;72(2):171–4.

70. Palumbo C, Pecoraro A, Knipper S, et al. Survival and complication rates of metastasectomy in patients with metastatic renal cell carcinoma treated exclusively with targeted therapy: a combined population-based analysis. Anticancer Res 2019;39(8):4357–61.

71. Joshi SS, Handorf EA, Zibelman M, et al. Treatment facility volume and survival in patients with metastatic renal cell carcinoma: a registry-based analysis. Eur Urol 2018;74(3):387–93.

72. Zaorsky NG, Lehrer EJ, Kothari G, et al. Stereotactic ablative radiation therapy for oligometastatic renal cell carcinoma (SABR ORCA): a meta-analysis of 28 studies. Eur Urol Oncol 2019;2(5):515–23.

73. Husain ZA, Sahgal A, De Salles A, et al. Stereotactic body radiotherapy for de novo spinal metastases: systematic review. J Neurosurg Spine 2017;27(3):295–302.

74. Welch BT, Callstrom MR, Morris JM, et al. Feasibility and oncologic control after percutaneous image guided ablation of metastatic renal cell carcinoma. J Urol 2014;192(2):357–63.

75. Maciolek KA, Abel EJ, Best S, et al. Percutaneous Microwave Ablation for Local Control of Metastatic Renal Cell Carcinoma. Abdom Radiology 2018 Sep;43(9):2446–54.

76. Geynisman DM, Hu JC, Liu L, et al. Treatment patterns and costs for metastatic renal cell carcinoma patients with private insurance in the United States. Clin Genitourin Cancer 2015;13(2):e93–100.

77. Cholley T, Thiery-Vuillemin A, Limat S, et al. Economic burden of metastatic clear-cell renal cell carcinoma for french patients treated with targeted therapies. Clin Genitourin Cancer 2019;17(1):e227–34.

78. Bang HJ, Littrup PJ, Goodrich DJ, et al. Percutaneous cryoablation of metastatic renal cell carcinoma for local tumor control: feasibility, outcomes, and estimated cost-effectiveness for palliation. J Vasc Interv Radiol 2012;23(6):770–7.

79. Murthy SC, Kim K, Rice TW, et al. Can we predict long-term survival after pulmonary metastasectomy for renal cell carcinoma? Ann Thorac Surg 2005;79(3):996–1003.

80. Kang MC, Kang CH, Lee HJ, et al. Accuracy of 16-channel multi-detector row chest computed tomography with thin sections in the detection of metastatic pulmonary nodules. Eur J Cardiothorac Surg 2008;33(3):473–9.

Minimally Invasive Surgery for Patients with Locally Advanced and/or Metastatic Renal Cell Carcinoma

Ezequiel Becher, MD*, Dora Jericevic, MD, William C. Huang, MD

KEYWORDS

- Minimally invasive surgery • Renal cell carcinoma • Metastatic renal cell carcinoma
- Advanced renal cell carcinoma • Robotic surgery • Nephrectomy

KEY POINTS

- Surgery continues to have a vital role in the management of advanced renal cell carcinoma.
- Minimally invasive surgery for localized renal cell carcinoma has been shown to provide comparable oncologic outcomes as open surgery, while decreasing treatment-related morbidity.
- With advances in technology and refinements in surgical technique, a minimally invasive surgical approach is feasible in select cases.
- Several high-volume centers have reported favorable interim oncologic and nononcologic outcomes using minimally invasive surgery, including cases with inferior vena cava involvement and regional adenopathy.
- Patient selection and surgeon experience are critical, as proper oncologic principles should never be compromised when utilizing a minimally invasive surgical approach.

INTRODUCTION

Radical nephrectomy (RN) is considered the preferred treatment of surgically resectable advanced renal cell carcinoma (aRCC) by most guidelines.[1–3] Open RN (ORN) can be a considerably morbid surgery, because it often entails a large incision, extensive bowel mobilization and elevated estimated blood loss (EBL), factors that translate into significant postoperative pain and a longer recovery. Minimally invasive surgery (MIS), whether performed laparoscopically or robotically, is well-established for localized tumors. MIS for localized tumors is associated with improved perioperative outcomes, while maintaining oncologic outcomes.[4–6] There is increasing evidence that MIS may be similarly beneficial in cases of aRCC.

This article discusses the role of MIS in the management of aRCC, highlighting the potential benefits and drawbacks. MIS approaches for inferior vena cava (IVC) thrombectomy and lymph node dissection (LND) are also covered. Additionally, we address the role of minimally invasive cytoreductive nephrectomy (CN) in the context of metastatic RCC (mRCC). For the purposes of this article, we define aRCC as stage cT2 disease or higher, given that large organ-confined disease may be technically challenging to extirpate and potentially difficult to distinguish from locally aRCC at diagnosis. Locally advanced disease encompasses patients with cT3 and cT4 disease with venous thrombi, extracapsular extension, adjacent organ involvement, and/or nodal disease.

Department of Urology, NYU Langone Health, 222 East 41st, 12th Floor, New York, NY 10017, USA
* Corresponding author.
E-mail address: Ezequiel.becher@nyulangone.org

Urol Clin N Am 47 (2020) 389–397
https://doi.org/10.1016/j.ucl.2020.04.004

HISTORY OF MINIMALLY INVASIVE SURGERY FOR RENAL MASSES

The first report of a laparoscopic kidney surgery dates to 1990 at Washington University by Dr Ralph Clayman's group.[7] The procedure was performed successfully in 6 hours and 45 minutes with a 300 mL EBL on an 85-year-old woman with a 3-cm midpole renal mass. She had an uncomplicated course and a 6-day length of stay. This successful procedure pioneered the way for significant advances in laparoscopic retroperitoneal surgery, with subsequent reports of laparoscopic partial nephrectomy and laparoscopic retroperitoneal LND (RPLND).[8]

Over the last decade, the increasing use of the robotic surgical platform has stimulated the adoption of MIS, thus contributing to the rising trend of nephron sparing surgery over RN.[9] With a flatter learning curve compared with laparoscopic surgery, along with other advantages such as the wristed instruments, 3-dimensional vision, and tremor suppression, surgeons have been emboldened to incorporate the minimally invasive approach for more complex scenarios, such as IVC invasion and local lymph node involvement.[10,11]

EVIDENCE AND POTENTIAL BENEFITS

When introducing any new technique in oncologic surgery, a primary concern is does the new method achieve at least the same oncologic efficacy as the established one? In this regard, several studies[4,6,12–14] support that for properly selected cases of aRCC, MIS can obtain equivalent overall survival, cancer-specific survival, and progression-free survival as open surgery. These studies also suggest that MIS for aRCC has similar benefits as those achieved with MIS for localized tumors, namely, equivalent oncologic control, with lower morbidity and shorter convalescence time.[4,6,12,13]

Using the Surveillance Epidemiology and End Results database and propensity score matching, Golombos and colleagues[13] compared the outcomes of MIS versus ORN. After a median follow-up of 57.1 months, they demonstrated comparable oncologic efficacy and superior perioperative outcomes in the MIS group. However, this article included all renal masses undergoing RN, 17% of which had tumors 7 cm or larger and 21% of which were stage III after matching.

Including only pT3a or higher tumors, Laird and colleagues[4] retrospectively analyzed matched cohorts of 25 laparoscopic RN (LRN) and 25 ORN cases with a median follow-up of 54.6 months. They observed that the MIS cohort had a statistically significant lower EBL (LRN 100 mL vs ORN 650 mL;

$P<.01$) and length of stay (LRN 4 days vs ORN 9 days; $P<.01$), while maintaining cancer-specific survival and progression-free survival.[4] A critique of this article is that the matched paired analysis may have underpowered the sample size, but its findings were replicated by a larger, nonmatched study from Bragayrac and colleagues.[6] Although there is substantial concordance among the studies,[6,12,14–16] the results remain limited to primarily level 3 and level 4 evidence.

In terms of perioperative outcomes, the benefit of lower EBL associated with the MIS approach is multifactorial, but is largely attributed to the pneumoperitoneum's homogeneous positive pressure applied to tissues during surgery. In vascular tumors such as clear cell RCC, this pneumoperitoneum is particularly beneficial in controlling bleeding from frail parasitic vessels, which often feed the tumor.

Perioperative outcomes are also important to note because a shorter convalescence may allow for potential improvements in survival. We know that surgery alone is not curative in many patients with aRCC. Subsequently those undergoing cytoreductive nephrectomy may have a delay in receipt of systemtic therapy. Additionally in patients with locally aRCC, a prolonged recovery may result in adjuvant therapy, particularly in clinical trials.[17] This particular aspect was highlighted by Gershman and colleagues[18] in their retrospective study evaluating factors contributing to the postoperative complications of 294 patients undergoing CN for M1 disease. On multivariate analysis, they found that undergoing MIS was independently associated with earlier administration of systemic therapy.[18]

Currently, several studies support the notion that minimally invasive RN can be safely performed even in more complex and clinically advanced cases. Depending on the study, the rates of Clavien grade IIIa or higher complications range from 3% to 10% for MIS, generally less than what is reported for ORN[12,19–22] (8%–25%).

ROBOTIC VERSUS LAPAROSCOPIC SURGERY

There are only a few studies comparing robotic RN (RRN) with LRN. In a multi-institutional retrospective study by Anele and colleagues,[23] the authors did not appreciate any significant differences in the perioperative outcomes of RRN versus LRN. Although, this study included patients undergoing RN for all tumor sizes, the proportion of patients with cT3 or higher disease, or undergoing CN, was higher in the robotic cohort, suggesting that surgeons may have tended to favor RRN over LRN when facing more complex cases. Despite its fairly large sample size (n = 941), further prospective randomized studies are warranted however, to draw stronger conclusions.

CASES OF RENAL VEIN AND/OR INFERIOR VENA CAVA INVOLVEMENT

The role of MIS in the management of patients with venous tumor thrombi (VTT) has significantly evolved since it was first described in 2003.[24] The latest reports demonstrate that indications for MIS have expanded to include level 3 and 4 tumor thrombi, extensive adenopathy along with disease in the chest resulting in a combined thoracic MIS approach.[10,25–27]

It is commonly accepted that Robot-assisted surgery is especially useful in cases with short tumor thrombi that either do not extend into the IVC (level 0) or do not extend far from the ostium such that they can be milked back (level 1). The robotic platform provides the surgeon with an enhanced ability to control these thrombi without the need for a cavotomy. However, most extensive level I thrombi require an incision into IVC. Techniques that replicate the use of the Satinsky clamp as a tangential clamp, allowing for a subsequent over-sewing of the removed vein ostium site without significantly interrupting IVC flow, as done in the open surgery approach, have been described.[28]

The management of more extensive tumor thrombi (level II–III) can also be done through a MIS approach. Chopra and colleagues[26] have described a reproducible step-by-step technique for the management of right and left sided level II to III IVC robotic thrombectomy and RRN. The authors suggest addressing the IVC first and mobilizing the kidney later, reportedly decreasing the risk of tumor embolization. After the IVC has been dissected and all lumbar veins have been identified, clipped, and divided, they proceed with the placement of Rummel tourniquets on the contralateral renal vein, as well as the IVC proximal and distal to the tumor borders. Next, they proceed with ligation of the renal artery and sequential cinching of the tourniquets. The unique step the authors describe is the transection of the thrombus-containing vein with a laparoscopic stapler. The authors state that this maneuver allows for a complete evaluation of the IVC's circumference and an early bagging of the thrombus once it is dissected, thus avoiding spillage. Even though the article suggests the technique can be used on level II and III thrombi, it does not address the concern of extensive liver mobilization required for some level III thrombi.

Wang and colleagues[25] have described their management of complex level III and IV tumor thrombi with a purely robotic approach, achieving

acceptable short- and medium-term oncologic outcomes. Even though there is substantial heterogeneity in complexity among their series of 13 patients, as well as concerns about the reproducibility of their technique, the authors should be congratulated on their pioneering efforts.

RETROPERITONEAL LYMPH NODE DISSECTION AND ADENOPATHY

The role of LND in aRCC is controversial. There is no high-level evidence that demonstrates a survival benefit of LND in aRCC.[29,30] However, LND seems to have an important role in staging patients with aRCC at the time of nephrectomy.[31] Even though these concepts are more thoroughly analyzed in another article in this issue (please see Pooja Unadkat and colleagues' artcile, "The Role of Lymphadenectomy in Patients with Advanced Renal Cell Carcinoma (RCC)," in this issue), we focus on the role of MIS in LND for aRCC.

Some studies suggest that MIS is associated with a less extensive or absent LND.[32–34] Although there is no clear oncologic benefit of LND in patients with aRCC (including those with clinically visible nodes), we do not advocate for the omission of a proper lymphadenectomy particularly in patients with suspicious nodes. The introduction and widespread use of robotic-assisted surgery has facilitated the performance of higher yield lymphadenectomies, achieving similar node counts as those seen with the open approach.[35]

There is no standardized lymphadenectomy template for RCC, given the lack of data supporting therapeutic benefit. This is not the case with nonseminomatous germ cell tumors (NSGCT) of the testis, where there are clear indications and quality metrics for RPLND. In this regard, Pearce and colleagues[36] have examined the clinical outcomes of robotic RPLND performed for NSGCT using a large multi-institutional series, concluding that robotic RPLND can achieve adequate oncologic metrics with an acceptable morbidity profile. Given that the most cephalad part of the RPLND template for NSGCT reaches the renal hilum, one could argue that part of the LND done for NSGCT mimics the LND done for aRCC. We cannot extrapolate the conclusions reached by Pearce and colleagues[36] to the RCC paradigm. The authors demonstrate that a meticulous and proper retroperitoenal lymph node dissection can be performed with low morbidity regardless of the primary site.

CRITIQUES AND POTENTIAL DRAWBACKS

One of the major concerns in oncologic MIS is the risk of tumor dissemination owing to the use of pneumoperitoneum in the setting of potentially aggressive tumor biology. There are reports of worsened oncologic outcomes and unusual sites of disease recurrence after MIS for various malignancies including cervical,[37] NSGCT,[38] and adrenocortical carcinoma.[39] In their prospective trial, Ramirez and colleagues[37] randomized women with early stage cervical carcinoma to open and MIS radical hysterectomy, observing that the MIS approach provided a lower cancer-specific survival and overall survival.

Incisional and local recurrences secondary to tumor spillage are rare phenomena in RCC,[40] accounting for less than 0.1% of cases (mostly described in case reports or series).[40–42] A meta-analysis comparing oncologic and perioperative outcomes of ORN and LRN was not able to find significant differences in overall local recurrence rates between these 2 approaches.[43] Even though this metanalysis included tumors of all sizes and stages, the recurrence rates were also comparable in the subgroup analysis of T3 and T4 tumors.[43] Song and colleagues[44] conducted a review of this subject, concluding that even though port site recurrence is rare, it entails a poor prognosis, with only 31% survival at 1 year in this small cohort (n = 16). However, no technical aspect was found to be a risk factor for occurrence of port site metastasis, suggesting that the tumor biology might play a greater role in the development of these unusual sites of recurrence.

In terms of local recurrence after RN, it is rare, accounting for 1% to 2% of open and MIS cases.[45] Resection of these isolated local recurrences has been shown to improve oncologic outcomes.[46,47] Some case series suggest that MIS is more advantageous than an open approach for the recurrence resection, achieving equivalent oncologic quality with lower morbidity.[45] However, the low prevalence of local recurrence makes it challenging to produce strong evidence to support the potential benefit of MIS in this setting.

The pneumoperitoneum system and inefficient bagging of the specimen are often considered putative causes of unusual site recurrence, including port sites.[44,48] However, there is no clear evidence that these are the causes of port site recurrences, and the rarity of this event makes it close to impossible to run any study to objectify this finding. Another potential risk factor for port site recurrence is specimen morcellation.[44] However, this procedure is now rarely used for RCC, mainly because it precludes standard pathologic examination of the specimen, thus limiting tumor staging.[49]

Regardless of the approach, adherence to strict oncologic principles is critical to minimize local recurrences. It is our belief, particularly for patients with aRCC, that careful manipulation of the mass without violation of tumor boundaries and an early bagging of the specimen are the key factors for mitigating unusual patterns of recurrence.

CYTOREDUCTIVE NEPHRECTOMY IN METASTATIC RENAL CELL CARCINOMA: A ROLE FOR MINIMALLY INVASIVE SURGERY?

In light of seminal clinical trials such as CARMENA and SURTIME, the role of CN in the context of mRCC is constantly being redefined.[50,51] Nevertheless, most guidelines agree that surgery plays an important role for the management of patients with mRCC who have a good performance status and do not present with poor risk features.[52]

A challenge yet to be fully explored is the impact of MIS for CN in the era of targeted therapy and immunotherapy. Several retrospective series report that the preoperative use of targeted molecular therapies (such as tyrosine kinase inhibitors) before CN does not increase the rate of perioperative complications.[53–55] Even though the study by Harshman and colleagues[55] did show the benefit of reduced EBL with MIS, only a minority of cases in this study were performed through a MIS approach. The SURTIME trial[51] randomized patients with mRCC and resectable primary tumors to either CN followed by systemic targeted therapy or CN preceded by systemic targeted therapy with progression as the primary endpoint. The safety of deferred CN was among the secondary end points. This trial did not find significant differences in perioperative morbidity of CN with prior targeted therapy, though it did not comment on surgical difficulty or approach (open vs MIS). Neither the retrospective series[55] nor the findings of SURTIME reported increased perioperative morbidity with the preoperative use of targeted therapy. However, the majority of these cases were performed through an open approach, which raises the concern of whether MIS is the right approach for these theoretically more difficult cases.

Regarding surgery after the use of immunotherapy, a series was recently published that describes the difficulty surgeons encountered when performing a CN in cases of complete distant response to immune checkpoint inhibitor therapy.[56] In their series of 11 patients (7 open and 4 MIS), they encountered serious intraoperative difficulties that resulted in longer median operative time procedures with an elevated average EBL (243 minutes and 903 mL, respectively). A history of immunotherapy should caution the surgeon that the case might be more difficult than expected and perhaps warrant an open approach. Until larger studies on these cases shine a brighter light on the matter, the approach chosen will have to be left to the discretion of the surgeon.

PROPER PATIENT SELECTION FOR MINIMALLY INVASIVE SURGERY IN ADVANCED RENAL CELL CARCINOMA

As previously mentioned, although MIS can achieve oncological results comparable to ORN, it does not imply that MIS is applicable to every patient scenario. It is important for surgeons to acknowledge their own level of expertise and comfort when selecting a surgical approach, keeping in mind that the proper approach will be one that derives the most benefit for the patient.

Proper patient selection cannot be driven solely on size or clinical stage. The current AJCC staging for RCC[57] describes cT2 tumors as confined to the kidney and 7 cm or larger, regardless of the maximum diameter. Tumors become cT3 if there is evidence of invasion either to the perirenal/sinus fat or to the segmental branches of the renal vein. Obviously, small cT3 tumors (vein thrombus or sinus fat involvement) may not be as technically challenging as a 7-cm left upper pole cT2 renal mass with large parasitic vessels and extensive regional adenopathy.

Even though clinical stage should not be the only driving factor in patient selection for MIS, it is still an important factor to consider, especially for more advanced stages. RN for tumors with invasion into neighboring organs can be extremely challenging. The largest retrospective series from experienced tertiary level institutions exploring surgical outcomes of nephrectomy in T4 disease report that the majority (if not all) of the cases were done through an open approach.[58–60] The series published by Oake and colleagues[60] does include cases performed laparoscopically (16%), which did not seem to be an indicator of adverse outcomes in the univariate analysis. However, it is important to add that invasion into neighboring organs (with concomitant organ resection) only accounted for 7.3% of the study population with the remaining categorized as T4 because of soft tissue invasion outside Gerota's fascia.

We have described the role and some technical aspects of MIS for IVC thrombectomy cases and LND. There are no clear patient selection criteria for a minimally invasive approach. The literature is filled with outcomes of complex cases performed minimally invasively that are certainly stimulating and a sign of progress. However, the enthusiasm should be met with caution and surgeons must always be aware of their limitations particularly as they pertain to novel treatment approaches.

NEW YORK UNIVERSITY EXPERIENCE ON MINIMALLY INVASIVE SURGERY FOR ADVANCED RENAL CELL CARCINOMA

At the department of Urology of New York University Langone Health, we began prospectively collecting the data on patients undergoing radical or partial nephrectomy for aRCC in 2004 as part of a prospectively maintained database including patients undergoing surgery for renal masses. This dataset captures our experience as we developed a formal program for robotic surgery.

During this period, from a total of 1668 patients, 302 (18%) had stage cT2 or higher disease. When examining all oncologic kidney surgery, the proportion performed for aRCC has been stable at approximately 20% over the last 16 years at our institution. However, we have observed an increasing percentage of our RNs being performed for aRCC (from 25% in 2006 to 70% in 2019; **Fig. 1**). This can be explained by an increasing

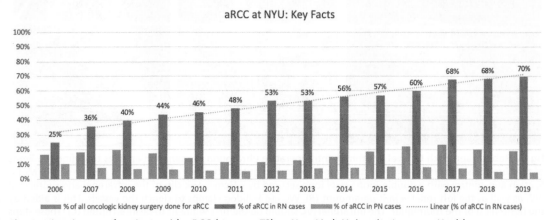

Fig. 1. Historic rate of patients with aRCC (stage ≥cT2) at New York University Langone Health.

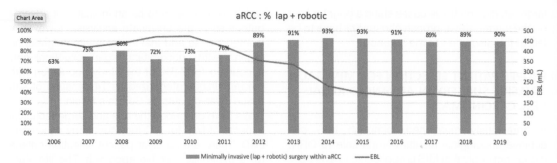

Fig. 2. Historic rate of patients undergoing MIS for aRCC (stage ≥cT2) at New York University Langone Health.

percentage of localized RCC being managed through partial nephrectomy instead of radical nephrectomy. Since 2012, MIS has constituted 90% of all oncologic kidney surgery, which has been associated with improvements in perioperative outcomes, such as EBL (from 450 mL in 2006–175 mL in 2019; **Fig. 2**).

With a thoughtful and stepwise application of MIS to our practice, we now incorporate a MIS approach in more complex cases of aRCC, such as those with IVC level I-II thrombi or regional adenopathy. At New York University, we routinely consider RRN with IVC thrombectomy for level I and II tumor thrombi. Our approach differs from what has been described elsewhere in this article in that we have not adopted the use of a stapler across the renal vein for level II thrombi. Our technique for level II thrombi consists of a venotomy either around the ostium of the renal vein (for short level II thrombi) or a cavotomy (for longer thrombi) with an intact extraction followed by an immediate bagging of the specimen (**Figs. 3 and 4**). With our

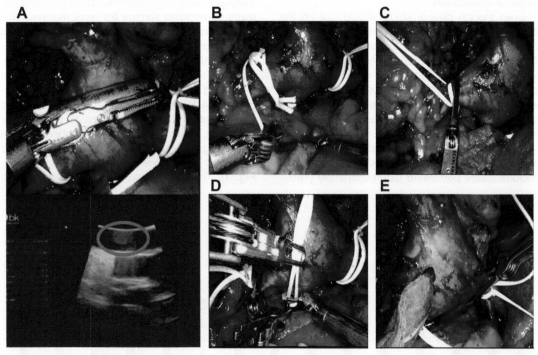

Fig. 3. Robotic approach to level II thrombi. Intraoperative ultrasound examination enables to define the limits of the thrombus (*red circle*), which in this case is extending outside the ostium of the right renal vein (*A*). Mobilization and control with a double-loop vessel loop secured by a Hem-o-Lok clip of the infrarenal and suprarenal IVC, as well as the left renal vein is paramount (*B*). We use bulldog clamps to clench the vessels. This is aided by the tightening of the tourniquet. The infrarenal IVC should be the first segment to be interrupted (*C*). These steps are repeated to close the circulation of the left renal vein (*D*) and suprarenal IVC (*E*), in that order.

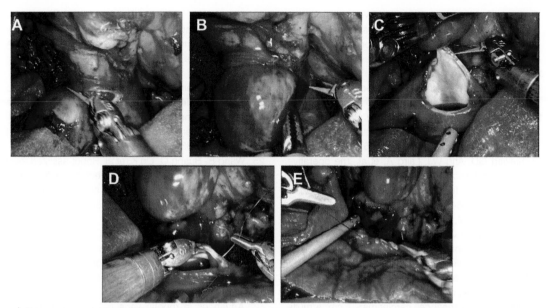

Fig. 4. IVC thrombectomy. After proper cinching of the tourniquets, a cavotomy on the anterior aspect of the IVC is made medial to the ostium of the right renal vein (*A*). The IVC is incised until a careful delivery of the tumor thrombus is done (*B*) (it is crucial to preserve the integrity of the tumor). The cavotomy is completed and the right renal vein containing the tumor is divided (*C*). A running 4-0 polypropylene suture is used to repair the IVC defect (*D, E*).

expanding experience of MIS RPLND in testis cancer, we are incorporating the same techniques for LND in patients with RCC.[61]

SUMMARY

In the era of targeted therapy and immunotherapy, surgery continues to have a role in the management of aRCC. Traditionally, cases of aRCC with IVC involvement or extensive adenopathy were performed through an open approach. However, advantages of the robotic platform have fostered the implementation of MIS in these more challenging scenarios. In properly selected patients, it seems that the MIS approach for aRCC provides comparable oncologic outcomes with decreased postoperative morbidity. Although MIS may not be applicable to all cases of aRCC, the role of MIS will continue to expand by adhering to proper oncologic principles and appropriate patient selection.

ACKNOWLEDGEMENTS

Dr Becher's fellowship program is funded by Intuitive Foundation.

REFERENCES

1. Ljungberg B, Albiges L, Abu-Ghanem Y, et al. European Association of Urology Guidelines on renal cell carcinoma: the 2019 update. Eur Urol 2019;75(5): 799–810.
2. Campbell S, Uzzo RG, Allaf ME, et al. Renal mass and localized renal cancer: AUA guideline. J Urol 2017;198(3):520–9.
3. Motzer RJ, Jonasch E, Michaelson MD, et al. NCCN guidelines insights: kidney cancer, version 2.2020. J Natl Compr Canc Netw 2019;17(11): 1278–85.
4. Laird A, Choy KC, Delaney H, et al. Matched pair analysis of laparoscopic versus open radical nephrectomy for the treatment of T3 renal cell carcinoma. World J Urol 2015;33(1):25–32.
5. Gill IS, Kavoussi LR, Lane BR, et al. Comparison of 1,800 laparoscopic and open partial nephrectomies for single renal tumors. J Urol 2007;178(1): 41–6.
6. Bragayrac LA, Abbotoy D, Attwood K, et al. Outcomes of minimal invasive vs open radical nephrectomy for the treatment of locally advanced renal-cell carcinoma. J Endourol 2016; 30(8):871–6.
7. Clayman RV, Kavoussi LR, Soper NJ, et al. Laparoscopic nephrectomy. N Engl J Med 1991;324(19): 1370–1.
8. Kerbl DC, McDougall EM, Clayman RV, et al. A history and evolution of laparoscopic nephrectomy: perspectives from the past and future directions in the surgical management of renal tumors. J Urol 2011;185(3):1150–4.

9. Patel HD, Mullins JK, Pierorazio PM, et al. Trends in renal surgery: robotic technology is associated with increased use of partial nephrectomy. J Urol 2013; 189(4):1229–35.

10. Gill IS, Metcalfe C, Abreu A, et al. Robotic level III inferior vena cava tumor thrombectomy: initial series. J Urol 2015;194(4):929–38.

11. Abaza R, Eun DD, Gallucci M, et al. Robotic surgery for renal cell carcinoma with vena caval tumor thrombus. Eur Urol Focus 2016;2(6):601–7.

12. Stewart GD, Ang WJ, Laird A, et al. The operative safety and oncological outcomes of laparoscopic nephrectomy for T3 renal cell cancer. BJU Int 2012;110(6):884–90.

13. Golombos DM, Chughtai B, Trinh QD, et al. Minimally invasive vs open nephrectomy in the modern era: does approach matter? World J Urol 2017; 35(10):1557–68.

14. Luciani LG, Porpiglia F, Cai T, et al. Operative safety and oncologic outcome of laparoscopic radical nephrectomy for renal cell carcinoma> 7 cm: a multicenter study of 222 patients. Urology 2013;81(6): 1239–45.

15. Ouellet S, Carmel M, Martel A, et al. Perioperative outcomes for laparoscopic radical nephrectomies performed on≥ 10 cm tumors. Can J Urol 2014; 21(5):7487–95.

16. Bragayrac LN, Hoffmeyer J, Abbotoy D, et al. Minimally invasive cytoreductive nephrectomy: a multi-institutional experience. World J Urol 2016;34(12): 1651–6.

17. Harshman LC, Drake CG, Haas NB, et al. Transforming the perioperative treatment paradigm in non-metastatic RCC—a possible path forward. Kidney Cancer 2017;1(1):31–40.

18. Gershman B, Moreira DM, Boorjian SA, et al. Comprehensive characterization of the perioperative morbidity of cytoreductive nephrectomy. Eur Urol 2016;69(1):84–91.

19. Bolton EM, Hennessy D, Lonergan PE, et al. Evaluating the perioperative safety of laparoscopic radical nephrectomy for large, non-metastatic renal tumours: a comparative analysis of T1-T2 with T3a tumours. Ir J Med Sci 2018;187(2):313–8.

20. Jackson BL, Fowler S, Williams ST, et al. Perioperative outcomes of cytoreductive nephrectomy in the UK in 2012. BJU Int 2015;116(6):905–10.

21. Petros FG, Angell JE, Abaza R. Outcomes of robotic nephrectomy including highest-complexity cases: largest series to date and literature review. Urology 2015;85(6):1352–8.

22. Ebbing J, Wiebach T, Kempkensteffen C, et al. Evaluation of perioperative complications in open and laparoscopic surgery for renal cell cancer with tumor thrombus involvement using the Clavien-Dindo classification. Eur J Surg Oncol 2015;41(7):941–52.

23. Anele UA, Marchioni M, Yang B, et al. Robotic versus laparoscopic radical nephrectomy: a large multi-institutional analysis (ROSULA Collaborative Group). World J Urol 2019;37(11): 2439–50.

24. Blute ML, Leibovich BC, Lohse CM, et al. The Mayo Clinic experience with surgical management, complications and outcome for patients with renal cell carcinoma and venous tumour thrombus. BJU Int 2004;94(1):33–41.

25. Wang B, Huang Q, Liu K, et al. Robot-assisted level III-IV inferior vena cava thrombectomy: initial series with step-by-step procedures and 1-yr outcomes. Eur Urol 2019. https://doi.org/10.1016/j.eururo. 2019.04.019.

26. Chopra S, Simone G, Metcalfe C, et al. Robot-assisted Level II-III inferior vena cava tumor thrombectomy: step-by-step technique and 1-year outcomes. Eur Urol 2017;72(2):267–74.

27. Kundavaram C, Abreu AL, Chopra S, et al. Advances in robotic vena cava tumor thrombectomy: intracaval balloon occlusion, patch grafting, and vena cavoscopy. Eur Urol 2016; 70(5):884–90.

28. Abaza R. Initial series of robotic radical nephrectomy with vena caval tumor thrombectomy. Eur Urol 2011;59(4):652–6.

29. Blom JH, van Poppel H, Marechal JM, et al. Radical nephrectomy with and without lymph-node dissection: final results of European Organization for Research and Treatment of Cancer (EORTC) randomized phase 3 trial 30881. Eur Urol 2009;55(1):28–34.

30. Bhindi B, Wallis CJD, Boorjian SA, et al. The role of lymph node dissection in the management of renal cell carcinoma: a systematic review and meta-analysis. BJU Int 2018;121(5):684–98.

31. Brito J 3rd, Gershman B. The role of lymph node dissection in the contemporary management of renal cell carcinoma: a critical appraisal of the evidence. Urol Oncol 2017;35(11):623–6.

32. Capitanio U, Stewart GD, Larcher A, et al. European temporal trends in the use of lymph node dissection in patients with renal cancer. Eur J Surg Oncol 2017; 43(11):2184–92.

33. Filson CP, Miller DC, Colt JS, et al. Surgical approach and the use of lymphadenectomy and adrenalectomy among patients undergoing radical nephrectomy for renal cell carcinoma. Urol Oncol 2012;30(6):856–63.

34. Osterberg EC, Golan S, Pes MPL, et al. International and multi-institutional assessment of factors associated with performance and quality of lymph node dissection during radical nephrectomy. Urology 2019;129:132–8.

35. Abaza R, Lowe G. Feasibility and adequacy of robot-assisted lymphadenectomy for renal-cell carcinoma. J Endourol 2011;25(7):1155–9.

36. Pearce SM, Golan S, Gorin MA, et al. Safety and early oncologic effectiveness of primary robotic retroperitoneal lymph node dissection for nonseminomatous germ cell testicular cancer. Eur Urol 2017;71(3):476–82.

37. Ramirez PT, Frumovitz M, Pareja R, et al. Minimally invasive versus abdominal radical hysterectomy for cervical cancer. N Engl J Med 2018;379(20):1895–904.

38. Calaway AC, Einhorn LH, Masterson TA, et al. Adverse surgical outcomes associated with robotic retroperitoneal lymph node dissection among patients with testicular cancer. Eur Urol 2019;76(5):607–9.

39. Miller BS, Gauger PG, Hammer GD, et al. Resection of adrenocortical carcinoma is less complete and local recurrence occurs sooner and more often after laparoscopic adrenalectomy than after open adrenalectomy. Surgery 2012;152(6):1150–7.

40. Tanaka K, Hara I, Takenaka A, et al. Incidence of local and port site recurrence of urologic cancer after laparoscopic surgery. Urology 2008;71(4):728–34.

41. Ploumidis A, Panoskaltsis T, Gavresea T, et al. Tumor seeding incidentally found two years after robotic-Assisted radical nephrectomy for papillary renal cell carcinoma. A case report and review of the literature. Int J Surg case Rep 2013;4(6):561–4.

42. Song JB, Tanagho YS, Kim EH, et al. Camera-port site metastasis of a renal-cell carcinoma after robot-assisted partial nephrectomy. J Endourol 2013;27(6):732–9.

43. Liu G, Ma Y, Wang S, et al. Laparoscopic versus open radical nephrectomy for renal cell carcinoma: a systematic review and meta-analysis. Transl Oncol 2017;10(4):501–10.

44. Song J, Kim E, Mobley J, et al. Port site metastasis after surgery for renal cell carcinoma: harbinger of future metastasis. J Urol 2014;192(2):364–8.

45. Yohannan J, Feng T, Berkowitz J, et al. Laparoscopic resection of local recurrence after previous radical nephrectomy for clinically localized renal-cell carcinoma: perioperative outcomes and initial observations. J endourology 2010; 24(10):1609–12.

46. Itano NB, Blute ML, Spotts B, et al. Outcome of isolated renal cell carcinoma fossa recurrence after nephrectomy. J Urol 2000;164(2):322–5.

47. Romeo A, Marchiñena PG, Jurado AM, et al. Renal fossa recurrence after radical nephrectomy: current management, and oncological outcomes. Urol Oncol. 2020 Feb;38(2):42.e7–42.e12. https://doi.org/10.1016/j.urolonc.2019.10.004. Epub 2019 Nov 9.

48. Kadi N, Isherwood M, Al-Akraa M, et al. Port-site metastasis after laparoscopic surgery for urological malignancy: forgotten or missed. Adv Urol 2012; 2012:609531.

49. Trpkov K, Grignon DJ, Bonsib SM, et al. Handling and staging of renal cell carcinoma: the International Society of Urological Pathology Consensus (ISUP) conference recommendations. Am J Surg Pathol 2013;37(10):1505–17.

50. Mejean A, Ravaud A, Thezenas S, et al. Sunitinib alone or after nephrectomy in metastatic renal-cell carcinoma. N Engl J Med 2018;379(5):417–27.

51. Bex A, Mulders P, Jewett M, et al. Comparison of immediate vs deferred cytoreductive nephrectomy in patients with synchronous metastatic renal cell carcinoma receiving sunitinib: the SURTIME randomized clinical trial. JAMA Oncol 2019;5(2):164–70.

52. Bex A, Albiges L, Ljungberg B, et al. Updated European association of urology guidelines for cytoreductive nephrectomy in patients with synchronous metastatic clear-cell renal cell carcinoma. Eur Urol 2018;74(6):805–9.

53. Margulis V, Matin SF, Tannir N, et al. Surgical morbidity associated with administration of targeted molecular therapies before cytoreductive nephrectomy or resection of locally recurrent renal cell carcinoma. J Urol 2008;180(1):94–8.

54. Thomas AA, Rini BI, Stephenson AJ, et al. Surgical resection of renal cell carcinoma after targeted therapy. J Urol 2009;182(3):881–6.

55. Harshman LC, Yu RJ, Allen GI, et al. Surgical outcomes and complications associated with presurgical tyrosine kinase inhibition for advanced renal cell carcinoma (RCC). Urol Oncol. 2013 Apr; 31(3):379–85. https://doi.org/10.1016/j.urolonc.2011.01.005. Epub 2011 Feb 25.

56. Pignot G, Thiery-Vuillemin A, Walz J, et al. Nephrectomy after complete response to immune checkpoint inhibitors for metastatic renal cell carcinoma: a new surgical challenge? Eur Urol 2020. https://doi.org/10.1016/j.eururo.2019.12.018.

57. Amin MB, Greene FL, Edge SB, et al. The eighth edition AJCC cancer staging manual: continuing to build a bridge from a population-based to a more "personalized" approach to cancer staging. CA Cancer J Clin 2017;67(2):93–9.

58. Borregales LD, Kim DY, Staller AL, et al. Prognosticators and outcomes of patients with renal cell carcinoma and adjacent organ invasion treated with radical nephrectomy. Urol Oncol 2016;34(5):237.e19-26.

59. Karellas ME, Jang TL, Kagiwada MA, et al. Advanced-stage renal cell carcinoma treated by radical nephrectomy and adjacent organ or structure resection. BJU Int 2009;103(2):160–4.

60. Oake JD, Patel P, Lavallee LT, et al. Outcomes and prognosticators of stage 4 renal cell carcinoma with pathological T4 primary lesion using a large Canadian multi-institutional database. Can Urol Assoc J 2019;14(2):24–30.

61. Taylor J, Becher E, Wysock JS, et al. Primary Robot-Assisted Retroperitoneal Lymph Node Dissectionfor Men with Non-Seminomatous Germ Cell Tumor: Experience from a Multi-Institutional Cohort, in press.

Radiation Therapy for Patients with Advanced Renal Cell Carcinoma

Joseph A. Miccio, MD[a], Oluwadamilola T. Oladeru, MD[b], Sung Jun Ma, MD[c], Kimberly L. Johung, MD, PhD[a],*

KEYWORDS

- Stereotactic radiosurgery • Stereotactic body radiation therapy • Renal cell carcinoma
- Radiotherapy

KEY POINTS

- The role of radiotherapy in advanced renal cell carcinoma has been increasing since the advent of high-dose-per-fraction treatment techniques.
- Excellent local control rates with minimal toxicity are possible with the use of stereotactic radiosurgery for intracranial metastases and stereotactic body radiation therapy (SBRT) for oligometastases to bone and visceral sites.
- Data are emerging supporting the efficacy and safety of SBRT as management of the primary tumor in select nonsurgical patients.
- Current research is focused on combining SBRT with immune checkpoint inhibitors in patients with metastatic renal cell carcinoma in an effort to potentiate the immune response and improve survival outcomes.

INTRODUCTION

Historically the role of radiotherapy (RT) in the management of renal cell carcinoma (RCC) was limited given several negative trials evaluating the effect of RT on survival in the neoadjuvant[1,2] and adjuvant[3,4] settings for patients with localized disease, and early in vitro studies reporting that RCC is a relatively radioresistant histology.[5] However, as higher-dose-per-fraction treatments became possible through the advent of stereotactic radiosurgery (SRS) for intracranial sites[6–9] and stereotactic body radiation therapy (SBRT; synonymous with stereotactic ablative RT) for extracranial sites,[8–15] there has been a resurgence of interest in RT for RCC. There are now published experiences showing the utility of RT in the treatment of RCC in a variety of clinical scenarios, including SBRT for RCC limited to the kidney,[13,16–24] SBRT for locally advanced (LA) RCC,[13,25–29] SRS for brain metastasis from RCC,[6–9] and SBRT for extracranial metastasis from RCC.[8–15] This article reviews the role of RT in patients with advanced RCC, including LA disease (≥T3 or >N0, M0) as well as metastatic RCC (mRCC), and ongoing efforts to optimize the incorporation of RT into the multimodality treatment paradigm for patients with mRCC to improve survival outcomes.

[a] Department of Therapeutic Radiology, Yale School of Medicine, 35 Park Street, New Haven, CT 06519, USA; [b] Harvard Radiation Oncology Program, Massachusetts General Hospital, Boston, MA, USA; [c] Department of Radiation Medicine, Roswell Park Comprehensive Cancer Center, Elm and Carlton Streets, Buffalo, NY 14263, USA
* Corresponding author.
E-mail address: Kimberly.johung@yale.edu

Urol Clin N Am 47 (2020) 399–411
https://doi.org/10.1016/j.ucl.2020.04.011
0094-0143/20/© 2020 Elsevier Inc. All rights reserved.

RADIOTHERAPY IN LOCALLY ADVANCED RENAL CELL CARCINOMA

Approximately 16% of patients with RCC present with LA, stage III disease.[30] Upfront radical nephrectomy remains the standard of care, followed by adjuvant sunitinib in select cases with clear cell histology.[31] However, recurrences after nephrectomy can be seen in up to 40% of LA RCC,[32] with a predominantly distant pattern of recurrence.[32] Treatment options for recurrent RCC include further surgery or radiation if local recurrence or systemic therapy.

RT has a limited role in LA RCC given the negative historical trials in this patient population. The role of neoadjuvant radiation therapy for surgical downstaging was investigated in the 1960s and 1970s, including 2 prospective clinical trials that compared neoadjuvant radiation therapy and upfront surgery. Both studies did not show an overall survival benefit at 5 years.[1,2] Similarly, the role of adjuvant radiation therapy was explored in 2 prospective clinical trials and failed to show a survival benefit, at least in part because of significant complication rates.[3,4] In a more recent meta-analysis including these trials and other retrospective studies, adjuvant radiation therapy was associated with a significant reduction in locoregional failure, but no survival benefit.[28] However, this analysis is limited by many of the included studies using outdated RT techniques and only a few studies being prospective. However, based on these data, current guidelines do not support routine fractionated radiation therapy in the neoadjuvant and adjuvant settings.

More recently, advanced radiation techniques have been evaluated in the treatment of RCC. Intraoperative radiation therapy (IORT) allows precise localization of the tumor bed while minimizing radiation dose to the surrounding normal organs. This approach was studied in multiple retrospective series,[33–35] the largest of which was a multicenter cohort of 98 patients, 71% of whom had T3 to T4 disease.[35] More than half of these patients received either neoadjuvant or adjuvant external beam RT, and 5-year disease-free survival was favorable compared with surgery alone, although in general isolated local recurrence is a rare event even in patients with LA RCC.[31] Given the lack of prospective evidence and no indication of an overall survival benefit, IORT is not routinely indicated in current guidelines.

Prospective data are emerging to support consideration of SBRT to the primary tumor as an option for patients with LA RCC who are not operable candidates. Treatment of the primary RCC tumor with SBRT is associated with excellent rates of local control for T1 to T2 lesions (local control rates of 70%–100% in a systematic review)[24] and thus has been gaining interest in recent years for early-stage disease.[36] However, extrapolation of this technique to LA RCC should be done with caution because it is not as well characterized in this patient population. One phase I dose escalation study included patients with up to T3 tumors, and none of the 15 patients with evaluable response had progressive disease, although outcomes for the subset with T3 tumors were not reported.[20] Most other prospective studies of SBRT for localized RCC did not report T stage,[17–19,21,22] although some of these studies did include tumors larger than 5 cm[18,22,23] and thus possibly some LA cases.

Data for SBRT specifically in T3 or greater tumors is largely restricted to reported outcomes in the small subset of LA patients included in some cohorts. In a dose escalation study of SBRT for RCC, 1 patient with T4 disease had local progression 11 months after treatment with SBRT (8 Gy in 5 fractions), which was successfully salvaged with repeat irradiation to the same dose and fractionation.[13] Three patients with T3 disease in 2 other studies showed no disease progression after follow-up of greater than 1 year.[25,26] The largest series of patients with LA tumors was published by Wang and colleagues,[27] who evaluated the efficacy of SBRT for patients with asynchronous bilateral RCC who previously had nephrectomy and developed a second primary in the contralateral kidney. Of the 4 patients with T3a tumors included, 3 had no local relapse at 3, 6, and 29 months of follow-up and 1 had local relapse at 12 months. One patient with T4 disease was included, who experienced local failure 6 months after treatment. However, the study is limited by its small fractionation size (3–5 Gy/fraction) with an extended fractionation scheme (10–17 fractions) and use of a gamma body irradiator.[27]

Although small retrospective and prospective studies are accumulating to support a role for SBRT to the primary tumor in early-stage RCC, data for patients with LA RCC are therefore limited, and the potential toxicities associated with treating these larger tumors have not been well described. Responses in the reported cases suggest that SBRT may provide a benefit in terms of local control and palliation of symptoms in LA RCC, although further studies are warranted.

RADIOTHERAPY IN METASTATIC RENAL CELL CARCINOMA
Management of Central Nervous System Metastasis

Although the rate of brain metastasis development in all patients with mRCC is approximately 2%, up to 16% of patients with thoracic and bone metastasis develop intracranial metastasis.[37] The development of brain metastases is associated with clear cell histology, sarcomatoid differentiation, larger tumor size, and node-positive disease at diagnosis.[38] In an epidemiologic evaluation of intracranial RT use in mRCC, the frequency of SRS use for brain metastasis from RCC increased from 27% in 2005 to 44% in 2014, and this trend was associated with improved overall survival.[39]

Local control rates with SRS for RCC brain metastasis are excellent, and generally approach or exceed 90% at 1 year (**Table 1**).[6–9,40–52] The largest study to date evaluating SRS for RCC brain metastasis is reported by Kano and colleagues,[45] who examined 531 lesions treated in 158 patients. With a median marginal dose of 18 Gy (range 10–22 Gy), the local control at 1 year was 87%, although survival at 1 year was only 38%. No studies are available evaluating survival of patients treated with SRS for RCC brain metastasis who are receiving modern systemic therapy (either ipilimumab/nivolumab or pembrolizumab/axitinib), but improved survival would be expected in this setting because most deaths in patients receiving radiosurgery for brain metastasis are attributable to non-neurologic causes, particularly for patients with limited (<4) brain metastasis.[53,54]

The use of focal therapy alone in the management of brain metastasis incurs the increased risk of distant intracranial failure compared with patients receiving whole-brain RT (WBRT).[53] In patients treated with single-fraction SRS or fractionated SRS, single metastasis and supratentorial location were associated with reduced risk of subsequent intracranial lesions.[55] For patients with a high intracranial disease burden, the benefit of additional whole-brain radiation in the setting of SRS has been suggested in select studies for patients with adequate performance status.[41,51] Despite this, given the cognitive sequelae of adding WBRT to SRS[56] and the success of salvage SRS,[57] WBRT is typically reserved for patients who cannot tolerate SRS or those with a high burden of intracranial disease or extensive intracranial relapse after initial SRS. Alternatively, for patients with a limited number of large, symptomatic, surgically accessible lesions, surgical metastasectomy with postoperative SRS can be considered for patients with good performance status.[58] For this patient population, preoperative SRS is an area of active study to reduce the rates of relapse with leptomeningeal disease after surgery and postoperative SRS.[59]

SRS for brain metastasis from mRCC is well tolerated, although there is evidence that SRS in combination with common systemic agents for SRS may increase toxicity. A series of 912 lesions treated with SRS showed that use of a tyrosine kinase inhibitor (TKI) within 30 days of SRS caused a significantly greater rate of radionecrosis (RN) (10.9% vs 6.4%),[60] although generally these rates are lower than the risk of RN in other series, which is reported to be approximately 17.2% at 1 year.[61] However, in combination with immune checkpoint inhibitors (ICIs), SRS carries a greater risk of symptomatic RN with a doubling of the incidence from 20% to 40% at approximately 3 years from treatment of patients on ICI.[62] Despite these risks, SRS for RCC is routine even in the setting of ICI given the excellent control rates and ability to control RN symptoms with supportive medications,[63] laser coagulation,[64] or surgery[65] for more severe cases.

SRS is an important tool in the management of brain metastasis from RCC. Most patients needing SRS have excellent local control with minimal toxicity. Surveillance MRI is warranted to assess for disease progression because distant intracranial failure requiring salvage therapy is common. Monitoring for neurologic symptoms after SRS is important for the early detection and treatment of RN, the rate of which is increased when combining SRS with TKI and especially ICI.

Spine Stereotactic Body Radiation Therapy

Bone is the second most common site of metastasis in patients with mRCC, with approximately 27% of patients diagnosed with bone metastasis at initial evaluation and 18% of patients with recurrent RCC recurring in the bone.[66,67] Among bone metastasis, the spine is the most frequently involved site,[66] with pain being the most frequently reported symptom.[68] Although surgery is indicated for select patients for spine stabilization, operative morbidity and complications with intraoperative blood loss may be significant.[69] Thus, SBRT is an alternate, noninvasive therapeutic tool that has shown promising local control rates with minimal toxicity in the prospective setting.[70–72]

One of the earliest prospective studies of SBRT for spine metastases from RCC evaluated single-fraction SBRT for 60 spine lesions, 70% of which were previously treated with conventional radiation therapy. With tumor doses ranging from 17.5 to 25 Gy in a single fraction and a median follow-up of 37 months, no radiation-induced toxicity was observed, 89% of lesions treated for pain (34 out of 38) had improvements in pain, and local control rate for tumors treated for radiographic progression was 88% (7 out of 8).[71] Similar outcomes were reported in a study by Nguyen and

Table 1
Studies evaluating stereotactic radiosurgery and stereotactic body radiation therapy in metastatic renal cell carcinoma

Author (Year)	Patients (Number of Lesions)	Sites Treated	Marginal Dose in Gy (Range)	Median Follow-up (mo)	1-y LC (%)	Toxicity
Schöggl et al,[88] 1998	23 (44)	Brain	Median 18 (8–30)	NR	NR (crude rate 100)	9% peritumoral edema 4% radionecrosis
Goyal et al,[41] 2000	29 (66)	Brain	Median 18 (7–24)	7	85	14% radiation necrosis
Payne et al,[47] 2000	21 (37)	Brain	Mean 20 (11–40)	NR	NR (crude rate 100)	0% radiation toxicity
Amendola et al,[40] 2000	22 (131)	Brain	Mean 18 (15–22); unknown whether marginal	NR	NR (crude rate 91)	5% radiation necrosis
Ikushima et al,[44] 2000	10 (24)	Brain	All 42 Gy in 7 fractions to isocenter	5	90	0% acute or late toxicity
Hernandez et al,[42] 2002	29 (92)	Brain	Median 17 (13–30)	7	100	NR
Hoshi et al,[43] 2002	42 (113)	Brain	Median 25 (20–30)	10	91	1 mortality secondary to tumor hemorrhage
Noel et al,[46] 2004	28 (65)	Brain	Median 17 (11–22) to isocenter	14	93	4% radionecrosis 4% seizure 4% tumor hemorrhage
Muacevic et al,[50] 2004	85 (376)	Brain	Median 21 (15–35)	11	94	4% grade V toxicity caused by tumor hemorrhage 13% symptomatic radiation toxicity
Samlowski et al,[48] 2008	32 (71)	Brain	NR (15–24)	NR	86	6% symptomatic radiation necrosis
Shuto et al,[49] 2010	105 (444)	Brain	Mean 22 (8–30)	7	71	2% tumor hemorrhage requiring surgery 5% peritumoral edema

Fokas et al,[51] 2010	68 (81)	Brain	Median 19 (15–22)	NR	83	2% grade III acute toxicity with SRS only, 3% with SRS + WBRT, overall 3% acute toxicity; 4% grade III late toxicity with SRS only, 5% with SRS + WBRT, overall 6% late toxicity
Kano et al,[45] 2011	158 (531)	Brain	Median 18 (10–22)	8	87	7% symptomatic adverse effects; 6% tumor hemorrhage
Staehler et al,[8] 2011	51 (135)	Brain	Median 20 (20–20)	16	100	4% grade II tumor hemorrhage; 6% grade II convulsions
Cochran et al,[6] 2012	61 (124)	Brain	Median 20 (13–24)	9	93	10% radiation-induced edema or necrosis; 3% hemorrhage
Kim et al,[89] 2012	46 (99)	Brain	Mean 21 (12–25)	NR	NR (crude rate 85)	2% symptomatic tumor hemorrhage; 2% hydrocephalus
Meyer et al,[52] 2018[a]	82 (120)	Brain	Median BED_3 75.1 Gy (SD 21.2)	13	82	Including extracranial metastasis; 50% grade I–II toxicity (asthenia, nausea, dyspnea, headache); 5% grade III toxicity (esophageal fistula, seizure, intratumoral hemorrhage, and increased ICP)
Stenman et al,[90] 2018[a]	31 (167)	Brain	Median 22 Gy (16.5–35.5)	63 (for all patients)	NR (crude rate 96)	NR for entire cohort; For all patients receiving targeted agents, 30% grade II–III toxicity (seizure, fatigue, pneumonitis most common)

(continued on next page)

Table 1
(continued)

Author (Year)	Patients (Number of Lesions)	Sites Treated	Marginal Dose in Gy (Range)	Median Follow-up (mo)	1-y LC (%)	Toxicity
Gerszten et al,[71] 2005	48 (60)	Spine	Mean 16 Gy in 1 fraction	37	96	0% radiation toxicity
Wersall et al,[80] 2005	50 (154)	117 lung, 6 adrenal gland, 12 kidney metastases, 5 thoracic wall, 4 bone, 3 mediastinum, 3 abdominal lymph gland, 2 liver, 1 spleen, 1 pancreas	Modal: 32 Gy in 4 fractions, 40 Gy in 4 fractions, and 45 Gy in 3 fractions	37	99	40% any toxicity 2% grade V toxicity
Svedman et al,[13] 2006	26 (77)	63 lung/mediastinum, 5 kidney metastases, 5 adrenal, 4 thoracic wall, 3 abdominal glands, 3 liver, 1 pelvis, 1 spleen	40 Gy in 4 fractions	52	100	58% grade I–II toxicity 4% Grade V toxicity
Teh et al,[14] 2007	14 (23)	Orbits, head and neck, lung, mediastinum, sternum, clavicle, scapula, humerus, rib, spine, abdominal wall	Modal 24 Gy in 3 fractions	9	81	No grade 2 or higher toxicity
Nguyen et al,[72] 2010	48 (55)	Spine	Modal 27 Gy in 3 fractions	13	80	No grade 3 or 4 neurologic toxicity 23% grade I fatigue 13% grade II fatigue 11% grade II nausea 7% grade II vomiting 2% grade III pain 2% grade III anemia
Staehler et al,[8] 2011	55 (105)	Spine	Median 20 Gy in 1 fraction	33	94	2% grade I abdominal pain
Balagamwala et al,[10] 2012	57 (88)	Spine	Median 15 Gy in 1 fraction (unknown whether marginal)	5	50	33% any toxicity 10.5% grade 1 fatigue 2% grade 3 nausea/vomiting 8% pain flare

Jhaveri et al,[11] 2012	18 (24)	14 spine, 4 ribs/clavicle, 6 pelvis	Modal 40 Gy in 5 fractions	10	NR	6% grade I toxicity
Zelefsky et al,[12] 2012	55 (105)	59 spine, 22 pelvic bones, 14 other, 9 femur, 1 lymph node	Modal 24 Gy in 1 fraction	12	72	4% grade 2 dermatitis, 7% fractures, 2% grade 4 erythema
Ranck et al,[81] 2013	18 (39)	11 bone, 10 abdominal lymph node, 7 mediastinum/hilum, 4 lung, 2 kidney metastases, 2 adrenal, 2 liver, 1 soft tissue	Modal 50 Gy in 10 fractions, (unknown whether marginal)	16	96	61% grade I fatigue, 11% grade 1 rib fracture, 6% grade 2 radiculitis, 6% grade 2 bone pain
Wang et al,[73] 2017	84 (184)	49 abdomen, 42 spine, 35 thorax, 25 nonspine, 16 soft tissue, 5 kidney, 3 spinal cord	Median 11 Gy in median 3 fractions	16	91	4% acute grade 3 toxicity (progressive pain and UTI) 2% late grade 3 toxicity (gastrointestinal bleed, compression fracture, and radiculopathy)
Meyer et al,[52] 2018[a]	109 (132)	75 spine, 11 nonspine bone and soft tissue, 46 visceral metastases	Median BED_3 90.6 Gy (SD 55.1) including brain metastasis	13	84	Including brain metastasis 50% grade I–II toxicity (asthenia, nausea, dyspnea, headache) 5% grade III toxicity (esophageal fistula, seizure, intratumoral hemorrhage, and increased ICP)
Stenman et al,[90] 2018[a]	65 (117)	68 lung, 18 lymph node, 7 adrenal, 5 kidney, 5 liver, 5 soft tissue, 4 bone, 4 local recurrence, 1 other	Modal 45 Gy in 3 fractions, unknown whether marginal)	63 (for all patients)	NR (crude rate 76)	NR for entire cohort For all patients receiving targeted agents, 30% grade II–III toxicity (seizure, fatigue, pneumonitis most common)
Franzese et al,[91] 2019	58 (73)	39 lungs, 19 lymph nodes, 7 bone, 5 adrenal, 3 liver	Median 45 Gy in 5 fractions	16	90	12% acute grade 1 toxicity (fatigue, pain, and nausea) 7% late grade 1–2 pneumonitis

Abbreviations: ICP, intracranial pressure; NR, not reported; SD, standard deviation; UTI, urinary tract infection; WBRT, whole-brain radiotherapy.

[a] Brain and extra–central nervous system metastases are reported in separate rows.

Adapted from Kothari G, Foroudi F, Gill S, Corcoran NM, Siva S. Outcomes of stereotactic radiotherapy for cranial and extracranial metastatic renal cell carcinoma: a systematic review. Acta Oncol. 2015;54(2):148-157 and Zaorsky NG, Lehrer EJ, Kothari G, Louie AV, Siva S. Stereotactic ablative radiation therapy for oligometastatic renal cell carcinoma (SABR ORCA): a meta-analysis of 28 studies. European Urology Oncology. 2019;2(5):515-523.

colleagues,[72] who evaluated outcomes after treatment of 55 spinal lesions with several SBRT regimens: 24 Gy in 1 fraction, 27 Gy in 3 fractions, or 30 Gy in 5 fractions. At 1 year, progression-free survival (PFS) was 82% with no high-grade neurologic toxicity observed, and there was pain resolution in 52% of patients. With the varying dose fractionation regimens of spine SBRT used in prior studies, 2 studies compared single versus multifraction regimens. A single fraction of 24 Gy had improved local control compared with single-fraction doses less than 24 Gy or multifraction regimens of 20 to 30 Gy in 3 to 5 fractions, attributed to a higher biologically effective dose (BED).[12,70] Additional retrospective studies provide evidence supporting spine SBRT for RCC with local control ranging from 72% to 96% at 1 year with differences primarily driven by dose and fractionation.[8,10,12,73] In addition, systemic therapy activity likely affects the efficacy of spine SBRT for RCC metastasis because 1 retrospective study reported an independent association of concurrent TKI with improved local control.[74]

In summary, SBRT is shown to be well tolerated with minimal toxicities and favorable outcomes in terms of pain relief and local control. Patient selection for spine SBRT is key, and ideal candidates have at least a 3-month life expectancy, adequate performance status, low epidural disease grade, with involvement of a maximum of 2 to 3 contiguous or noncontiguous spinal segments, no frank spinal cord compression, and the ability to lie flat and tolerate the treatment.[75] For patients who are not candidates for SBRT but may benefit from palliative treatment of spinal metastasis, conventionally fractionated RT (ie, 30 Gy in 10 fractions) can be delivered, although this treatment strategy is less effective than SBRT.[76]

Management of Other Sites of Metastatic Disease

Outside of the central nervous system and spine, RT has a role in the palliation and local control of RCC metastasis to bone and visceral sites, and as well as treatment of the primary tumor in patients with mRCC. Patients with pain from RCC skeletal metastasis have been shown to have significant pain response to both fractionated RT[77] and SBRT.[78] A phase II trial of palliative RT for mRCC treated 24 patients for bone pain to 30 Gy in 10 fractions and showed that 83% of patients experienced site-specific pain relief after RT, although with a varied duration of response (median 3 months, range 1–15 months). However, this study may be limited because, since the time of publication in 2005, more effective systemic

regimens have emerged which may affect local control and thus pain response. A more recent study from 2018 retrospectively reviewed outcomes of patients with skeletal metastasis from RCC treated with fractionated RT, mostly 30 Gy in 10 fractions. Fifty-three sites were palliated in 40 total patients, with pain control achieved in 73.6% of lesions with a median duration of pain response of 22.9 months.[77]

More recently, SBRT has been evaluated in the palliation and local control of painful bone metastases. The biological rationale for this makes particular sense for RCC, because historical in vitro studies showed relative radioresistance of RCC[5] and a retrospective review showed increased pain response rates with higher BED.[79] A retrospective review comparing patients receiving either SBRT (most common dose 27 Gy in 3 fractions) or fractionated RT (most common dose 20 Gy in 5 fractions) to painful bony metastasis from RCC showed greater efficacy with SBRT. Symptom control rates were approximately twice as high and more durable for patients receiving SBRT versus fractionated RT, with 1-year rates of 74.9% versus 39.9% and 2-year rates of 74.9% versus 35.7%. Furthermore, on multivariable analysis, BED greater than or equal to 80 was significantly associated with improved clinical response, radiographic response, and local control.[78] These results are corroborated by another report showing high BED (in this case >85 Gy) leading to faster and more durable pain relief compared with lower BED.[11]

SBRT has also proved effective for the management of visceral metastases from RCC, with a prospective study evaluating 77 target lesions showing 100% local control at 1 year with minimal toxicity.[13] Additional retrospective reviews of SBRT in this setting have shown relief of pain correlating to the treated metastatic sites and local control of 72% to 99% at 1 year.[12,14,80–82]

There have been several studies evaluating SBRT to the primary tumor in patients with mRCC as well. One study retrospectively reviewed the outcomes of SBRT to the primary tumor in patients with RCC and included 6 patients with mRCC.[26] The local control was reported to be 100%, but the rationale for treating these patients was not reported; presumably the patients were symptomatic with pain and/or hematuria. The investigators do report that all 4 patients in this series that had flank pain and/or hematuria before RT had resolution of their symptoms after RT, suggesting a palliative benefit to SBRT for LA disease in select patients. A pilot study from Roswell Park Cancer Institute examined cytoreductive nephrectomy specimens after neoadjuvant SBRT in patients with mRCC. Compared with archived RCC tumors without neoadjuvant RT, the SBRT-treated tumors had evidence of immunomodulation with higher expression of calreticulin and tumor-associated antigens, and a higher percentage of proliferating T cells.[83] These data suggest that SBRT to the primary RCC tumor in patients with mRCC has the potential to affect the efficacy of immunotherapeutic agents given this altered tumor microenvironment.

COMBINATION OF RADIOTHERAPY WITH SYSTEMIC THERAPY AND FUTURE DIRECTIONS

It is clear that RT has a role in palliation of LA RCC and mRCC, and that SBRT and SRS have the ability to provide excellent local control to the primary tumor as well as metastatic sites with limited toxicity. However, strategies to optimally combine RT with systemic therapy in an effort to improve survival outcomes is a topic of active study. The current efforts can be conceptually broken down into 2 scenarios: treatment of oligometastatic patients (typically with 1–5 total sites of disease) and treatment of oligoprogressive patients (typically with 1–5 progressing sites of disease with any number of metastases). In patients with oligoprogressive disease, SBRT is being evaluated as a noninvasive measure of eliminating clones that have become resistant to systemic therapy. In patients with oligometastatic disease, SBRT has been evaluated as a way to defer systemic therapy and/or improve PFS.

Table 2
Current trials involving immunotherapy in combination with stereotactic body radiation therapy in metastatic renal cell carcinoma

NCT Number	Study Phase	SBRT Dose and Fractionation	Intervention in Combination with SBRT	Estimated Enrollment	Expected Primary Completion Date
NCT01896271	Single-arm phase II	8–20 Gy in 1–3 fractions	High-dose IL-2	26	12/2019
NCT02306954	Randomized phase II	40 Gy in 2 fractions	High-dose IL-2	84	01/2020
NCT01884961	Single-arm phase II	18–36 Gy in 3 fractions	High-dose IL-2	35	06/2019
NCT03474497	Single-arm phase II	24 Gy in 3 fractions	Intralesional IL-2 and pembrolizumab	45	07/2021
NCT03065179	Single-arm phase II	Not specified	Ipilimumab and nivolumab	25	01/2020
NCT02781506	Single-arm phase II	Dose not specified, 1–3 fractions	Nivolumab	87	12/2020
NCT02855203	phase I/II	18–20 Gy in 1 fraction	Pembrolizumab	30	07/2020
NCT02318771	phase I	20 Gy in 5 fractions or 8 Gy in 1 fraction	Pembrolizumab	40	12/2019
NCT02599779	phase II	Not specified	Pembrolizumab	25	03/2020
NCT03115801	Randomized phase II	30 Gy in 3 fractions	Nivolumab	112	12/2020
NCT03511391	Randomized phase II	24 Gy in 3 fractions	Pembrolizumab or nivolumab	97	02/2022
NCT03050060	Single-arm phase II	Not specified	Nelfinavir and pembrolizumab, nivolumab, or atezolizumab	120	12/2021

Abbreviations: IL, interleukin; NCT, National Clinical Trial.

One major study from the Groupe d'étude des tumeurs urogénitales (GETUG) retrospectively evaluated the outcomes of 188 oligometastatic and oligoprogressive patients with mRCC treated with SBRT to 1 to 5 sites. A total of 101 patients received SBRT for oligoprogressive mRCC, mostly while on first-line therapy with TKIs, and these patients showed a median PFS of 8.6 months from the time of SBRT to all sites of progression. The 63 patients who presented with oligometastatic disease were treated exclusively with SBRT and no systemic therapy; approximately one-third of these patients did not relapse at the end of follow-up (median follow-up of 15 months), with a median time to systemic therapy initiation of 14.2 months.[52] In line with this are findings from Zhang and colleagues,[84] where SBRT was used to defer systemic therapy in patients with oligometastatic RCC. In their retrospective review of a prospective database, 47 patients were identified, ~75% of whom had a single site of metastatic disease, most commonly to bone. The median time from SBRT to the start of systemic therapy was 15.2 months, and almost 40% of patients received no systemic therapy and were alive after SBRT at a median follow-up of 25 months.[84]

These promising studies show that, for select patients with mRCC, it is possible that aggressive local therapy can delay systemic therapy for treatment-naive patients and prevent changing systemic therapy in patients with oligoprogressive disease who may still be experiencing systemic benefit from their current therapy. Compared with other forms of local therapy, such as surgery and thermal ablation techniques, SBRT is noninvasive and causes minimal, if any, delay in the systemic therapy schedule, which remains the backbone of therapy for patients with widely metastatic disease.

Because 2 first-line systemic regimens for mRCC now include ICI (combination ipilimumab/nivolumab and pembrolizumab/axitinib), many groups are interested in combining SBRT with ICI to evaluate whether SBRT can potentiate the systemic response to immunotherapy given the known immunomodulatory effects of SBRT[83] and reports on abscopal response in patients with mRCC treated with RT.[85,86] There have been more than a dozen trials initiated combining SBRT with ICI and other immuno-oncology agents in patients with mRCC,[87] which are described in **Table 2**. The results of these trials are awaited to help define the utility of SBRT in combination with ICI for patients with mRCC.

SUMMARY

With the advent of high-dose-per-fraction RT techniques, namely SRS and SBRT, the role of RT in RCC is increasing. RT can be considered for palliation and local control of patients with LA RCC tumors who are not operative candidates, as well as palliation and local control of intracranial and extracranial metastases. Current research is focused on the use of SBRT in patients receiving immunotherapeutic agents in an effort to improve survival outcomes.

REFERENCES

1. van der Werf-Messing B. Carcinoma of the kidney. Cancer 1973;32(5):1056–61.
2. Juusela H, Malmio K, Alfthan O, et al. Preoperative irradiation in the treatment of renal adenocarcinoma. Scand J Urol Nephrol 1977;11(3):277–81.
3. Finney R. The value of radiotherapy in the treatment of hypernephroma–a clinical trial. Br J Urol 1973; 45(3):258–69.
4. Kjaer M, Iversen P, Hvidt V, et al. A randomized trial of postoperative radiotherapy versus observation in stage II and III renal adenocarcinoma. A study by the Copenhagen Renal Cancer Study Group. Scand J Urol Nephrol 1987; 21(4):285–9.
5. Deschavanne PJ, Fertil B. A review of human cell radiosensitivity in vitro. Int J Radiat Oncol Biol Phys 1996;34(1):251–66.
6. Cochran DC, Chan MD, Aklilu M, et al. The effect of targeted agents on outcomes in patients with brain metastases from renal cell carcinoma treated with Gamma Knife surgery. J Neurosurg 2012;116(5): 978–83.
7. Kim YH, Kim JW, Chung HT, et al. Brain metastasis from renal cell carcinoma. Prog Neurol Surg 2012; 25:163–75.
8. Staehler M, Haseke N, Nuhn P, et al. Simultaneous anti-angiogenic therapy and single-fraction radiosurgery in clinically relevant metastases from renal cell carcinoma. BJU Int 2011;108(5):673–8.
9. Kothari G, Foroudi F, Gill S, et al. Outcomes of stereotactic radiotherapy for cranial and extracranial metastatic renal cell carcinoma: a systematic review. Acta Oncol 2015;54(2):148–57.
10. Balagamwala EH, Angelov L, Koyfman SA, et al. Single-fraction stereotactic body radiotherapy for spinal metastases from renal cell carcinoma. J Neurosurg Spine 2012;17(6):556–64.
11. Jhaveri PM, Teh BS, Paulino AC, et al. A dose-response relationship for time to bone pain resolution after stereotactic body radiotherapy (SBRT) for renal cell carcinoma (RCC) bony metastases. Acta Oncol 2012;51(5):584–8.

12. Zelefsky MJ, Greco C, Motzer R, et al. Tumor control outcomes after hypofractionated and single-dose stereotactic image-guided intensity-modulated radiotherapy for extracranial metastases from renal cell carcinoma. Int J Radiat Oncol Biol Phys 2012; 82(5):1744–8.

13. Svedman C, Sandstrom P, Pisa P, et al. A prospective Phase II trial of using extracranial stereotactic radiotherapy in primary and metastatic renal cell carcinoma. Acta Oncol 2006;45(7):870–5.

14. Teh B, Bloch C, Galli-Guevara M, et al. The treatment of primary and metastatic renal cell carcinoma (RCC) with image-guided stereotactic body radiation therapy (SBRT). Biomed Imaging Interv J 2007;3(1):e6.

15. Corbin KS, Ranck MC, Hasselle MD, et al. Feasibility and toxicity of hypofractionated image guided radiation therapy for large volume limited metastatic disease. Pract Radiat Oncol 2013;3(4):316–22.

16. Miccio J, Johung K. When surgery is not an option in renal cell carcinoma: the evolving role of stereotactic body radiation therapy. Oncology (Williston Park) 2019;33(5):167–73, 177.

17. Staehler M, Bader M, Schlenker B, et al. Single fraction radiosurgery for the treatment of renal tumors. J Urol 2015;193(3):771–5.

18. Siva S, Pham DJ, Tan TH, et al. Principal analysis of a phase ib trial of stereotactic body radiation therapy (SBRT) for primary kidney cancer. Int J Radiat Oncol Biol Phys 2016;96(2):S96.

19. McBride SM, Wagner AA, Kaplan ID. A phase 1 dose-escalation study of robotic radiosurgery in inoperable primary renal cancer. Int J Radiat Oncol Biol Phys 2013;87(2):S84.

20. Ponsky L, Lo SS, Zhang Y, et al. Phase I dose-escalation study of stereotactic body radiotherapy (SBRT) for poor surgical candidates with localized renal cell carcinoma. Radiother Oncol 2015;117(1):183–7.

21. Kaplan ID, Redrosa I, Martin C, et al. Results of a Phase I Dose Escalation Study of Stereotactic Radiosurgery for Primary Renal Tumors. Int J Radiat Oncol Biol Phys 2010;78(3):S191.

22. Pham D, Thompson A, Kron T, et al. Stereotactic ablative body radiation therapy for primary kidney cancer: a 3-dimensional conformal technique associated with low rates of early toxicity. Int J Radiat Oncol Biol Phys 2014;90(5):1061–8.

23. Siva S, Pham D, Kron T, et al. Stereotactic ablative body radiotherapy for inoperable primary kidney cancer: a prospective clinical trial. BJU Int 2017; 120(5):623–30.

24. Correa RJM, Louie AV, Zaorsky NG, et al. The emerging role of stereotactic ablative radiotherapy for primary renal cell carcinoma: a systematic review and meta-analysis. Eur Urol Focus 2019;5(6):958–69.

25. Kaidar-Person O, Price A, Schreiber E, et al. Stereotactic body radiotherapy for large primary renal cell carcinoma. Clin Genitourin Cancer 2017;15(5):e851–4.

26. Chang JH, Cheung P, Erler D, et al. Stereotactic ablative body radiotherapy for primary renal cell carcinoma in non-surgical candidates: initial clinical experience. Clin Oncol 2016;28(9):e109–14.

27. Wang YJ, Han TT, Xue JX, et al. Stereotactic gamma-ray body radiation therapy for asynchronous bilateral renal cell carcinoma. Radiol Med 2014;119(11):878–83.

28. Tunio MA, Hashmi A, Rafi M. Need for a new trial to evaluate postoperative radiotherapy in renal cell carcinoma: a meta-analysis of randomized controlled trials. Ann Oncol 2010;21(9):1839–45.

29. Nikolaev A, Benda R. Palliative radiation therapy for symptomatic control of inoperable renal cell carcinoma. Urol Case Rep 2015;4:51–2.

30. Surveillance E, and End Results Program. Cancer Stat FActs: Kidney and Renal Pelvis Cancer. 2019. Available at: https://seer.cancer.gov/statfacts/html/kidrp.html. Accessed November 25, 2019.

31. Otaibi MA, Tanguay S. Locally advanced renal cell carcinoma. Can Urol Assoc J 2007;1(2 Suppl):S55–61.

32. Janzen NK, Kim HL, Figlin RA, et al. Surveillance after radical or partial nephrectomy for localized renal cell carcinoma and management of recurrent disease. Urol Clin North Am 2003;30(4):843–52.

33. Pilar A, Gupta M, Ghosh Laskar S, et al. Intraoperative radiotherapy: review of techniques and results. Ecancermedicalscience 2017;11:750.

34. Calvo FA, Sole CV, Martinez-Monge R, et al. Intraoperative EBRT and resection for renal cell carcinoma: twenty-year outcomes. Strahlenther Onkol 2013;189(2):129–36.

35. Paly JJ, Hallemeier CL, Biggs PJ, et al. Outcomes in a multi-institutional cohort of patients treated with intraoperative radiation therapy for advanced or recurrent renal cell carcinoma. Int J Radiat Oncol Biol Phys 2014;88(3):618–23.

36. Wegner RE, Abel S, Vemana G, et al. Utilization of stereotactic ablative body radiation therapy for intact renal cell carcinoma: trends in treatment and predictors of outcome. Adv Radiat Oncol 2019; 5(1):85–91.

37. Bianchi M, Sun M, Jeldres C, et al. Distribution of metastatic sites in renal cell carcinoma: a population-based analysis. Ann Oncol 2011;23(4):973–80.

38. Sun M, De Velasco G, Brastianos PK, et al. The development of brain metastases in patients with renal cell carcinoma: epidemiologic trends, survival, and clinical risk factors using a population-based cohort. Eur Urol Focus 2019;5(3):474–81.

39. Haque W, Verma V, Butler EB, et al. Utilization of stereotactic radiosurgery for renal cell carcinoma brain

metastases. Clin Genitourin Cancer 2018;16(4): e935–43.

40. Amendola BE, Wolf AL, Coy SR, et al. Brain metastases in renal cell carcinoma: management with gamma knife radiosurgery. Cancer J 2000;6(6): 372–6.

41. Goyal LK, Suh JH, Reddy CA, et al. The role of whole brain radiotherapy and stereotactic radiosurgery on brain metastases from renal cell carcinoma. Int J Radiat Oncol Biol Phys 2000;47(4):1007–12.

42. Hernandez L, Zamorano L, Sloan A, et al. Gamma knife radiosurgery for renal cell carcinoma brain metastases. J Neurosurg 2002;97(5 Suppl): 489–93.

43. Hoshi S, Jokura H, Nakamura H, et al. Gamma-knife radiosurgery for brain metastasis of renal cell carcinoma: Results in 42 patients. Int J Urol 2002;9(11): 618–25.

44. Ikushima H, Tokuuye K, Sumi M, et al. Fractionated stereotactic radiotherapy of brain metastases from renal cell carcinoma. Int J Radiat Oncol Biol Phys 2000;48(5):1389–93.

45. Kano H, Iyer A, Kondziolka D, et al. Outcome predictors of gamma knife radiosurgery for renal cell carcinoma metastases. Neurosurgery 2011;69(6): 1232–9.

46. Noel G, Valery CA, Boisserie G, et al. LINAC radiosurgery for brain metastasis of renal cell carcinoma. Urol Oncol 2004;22(1):25–31.

47. Payne BR, Prasad D, Szeifert G, et al. Gamma surgery for intracranial metastases from renal cell carcinoma. J Neurosurg 2000;92(5):760–5.

48. Samlowski WE, Majer M, Boucher KM, et al. Multidisciplinary treatment of brain metastases derived from clear cell renal cancer incorporating stereotactic radiosurgery. Cancer 2008;113(9):2539–48.

49. Shuto T, Matsunaga S, Suenaga J, et al. Treatment strategy for metastatic brain tumors from renal cell carcinoma: selection of gamma knife surgery or craniotomy for control of growth and peritumoral edema. J Neurooncol 2010;98(2):169–75.

50. Muacevic A, Kreth FW, Mack A, et al. Stereotactic radiosurgery without radiation therapy providing high local tumor control of multiple brain metastases from renal cell carcinoma. Minim Invasive Neurosurg 2004;47(4):203–8.

51. Fokas E, Henzel M, Hamm K, et al. Radiotherapy for brain metastases from renal cell cancer: should whole-brain radiotherapy be added to stereotactic radiosurgery?: analysis of 88 patients. Strahlenther Onkol 2010;186(4):210–7.

52. Meyer E, Pasquier D, Bernadou G, et al. Stereotactic radiation therapy in the strategy of treatment of metastatic renal cell carcinoma: A study of the Getug group. Eur J Cancer 2018;98:38–47.

53. Kocher M, Soffietti R, Abacioglu U, et al. Adjuvant whole-brain radiotherapy versus observation after radiosurgery or surgical resection of one to three cerebral metastases: results of the EORTC 22952-26001 study. J Clin Oncol 2011;29(2):134–41.

54. McTyre ER, Johnson AG, Ruiz J, et al. Predictors of neurologic and nonneurologic death in patients with brain metastasis initially treated with upfront stereotactic radiosurgery without whole-brain radiation therapy. Neuro Oncol 2017;19(4):558–66.

55. Rades D, Dziggel L, Blanck O, et al. Predicting the risk of developing new cerebral lesions after stereotactic radiosurgery or fractionated stereotactic radiotherapy for brain metastases from renal cell carcinoma. Anticancer Res 2018;38(5):2973–6.

56. Brown PD, Jaeckle K, Ballman KV, et al. Effect of radiosurgery alone vs radiosurgery with whole brain radiation therapy on cognitive function in patients with 1 to 3 brain metastases: a randomized clinical TrialSRS with or without WBRT and cognitive function in patients with brain MetastasesSRS with or without WBRT and cognitive function in patients with brain metastases. JAMA 2016;316(4):401–9.

57. Fritz C, Borsky K, Stark LS, et al. Repeated courses of radiosurgery for new brain metastases to defer whole brain radiotherapy: feasibility and outcome with validation of the new prognostic metric brain metastasis velocity. Front Oncol 2018;8:551.

58. Choi CY, Chang SD, Gibbs IC, et al. Stereotactic radiosurgery of the postoperative resection cavity for brain metastases: prospective evaluation of target margin on tumor control. Int J Radiat Oncol Biol Phys 2012;84(2):336–42.

59. Prabhu RS, Patel KR, Press RH, et al. Preoperative vs postoperative radiosurgery for resected brain metastases: a review. Neurosurgery 2018;84(1): 19–29.

60. Juloori A, Miller JA, Parsai S, et al. Overall survival and response to radiation and targeted therapies among patients with renal cell carcinoma brain metastases. J Neurosurg 2019;1–9. https://doi.org/10.3171/2018.8.JNS182100.

61. Kohutek ZA, Yamada Y, Chan TA, et al. Long-term risk of radionecrosis and imaging changes after stereotactic radiosurgery for brain metastases. J Neurooncol 2015;125(1):149–56.

62. Martin AM, Cagney DN, Catalano PJ, et al. Immunotherapy and symptomatic radiation necrosis in patients with brain metastases treated with stereotactic radiation. JAMA Oncol 2018;4(8): 1123–4.

63. Vellayappan B, Tan CL, Yong C, et al. Diagnosis and management of radiation necrosis in patients with brain metastases. Front Oncol 2018;8:395.

64. Sharma M, Balasubramanian S, Silva D, et al. Laser interstitial thermal therapy in the management of brain metastasis and radiation necrosis after radiosurgery: An overview. Expert Rev Neurother 2016; 16(2):223–32.

65. Patel U, Patel A, Cobb C, et al. The management of brain necrosis as a result of SRS treatment for intracranial tumors. Transl Cancer Res 2014;3(4):373–82.

66. Swanson DA, Orovan WL, Johnson DE, et al. Osseous metastases secondary to renal cell carcinoma. Urology 1981;18(6):556–61.

67. Levy DA, Slaton JW, Swanson DA, et al. Stage specific guidelines for surveillance after radical nephrectomy for local renal cell carcinoma. J Urol 1998;159(4):1163–7.

68. Kassamali RH, Ganeshan A, Hoey ETD, et al. Pain management in spinal metastases: the role of percutaneous vertebral augmentation. Ann Oncol 2010; 22(4):782–6.

69. Sundaresan N, Choi IS, Hughes JE, et al. Treatment of spinal metastases from kidney cancer by presurgical embolization and resection. J Neurosurg 1990; 73(4):548–54.

70. Ghia AJ, Chang EL, Bishop AJ, et al. Single-fraction versus multifraction spinal stereotactic radiosurgery for spinal metastases from renal cell carcinoma: secondary analysis of Phase I/II trials. J Neurosurg Spine 2016;24(5):829–36.

71. Gerszten PC, Burton SA, Ozhasoglu C, et al. Stereotactic radiosurgery for spinal metastases from renal cell carcinoma. J Neurosurg Spine 2005;3(4): 288–95.

72. Nguyen QN, Shiu AS, Rhines LD, et al. Management of spinal metastases from renal cell carcinoma using stereotactic body radiotherapy. Int J Radiat Oncol Biol Phys 2010;76(4):1185–92.

73. Wang CJ, Christie A, Lin MH, et al. Safety and efficacy of stereotactic ablative radiation therapy for renal cell carcinoma extracranial metastases. Int J Radiat Oncol Biol Phys 2017;98(1):91–100.

74. Miller JA, Balagamwala EH, Angelov L, et al. Spine stereotactic radiosurgery with concurrent tyrosine kinase inhibitors for metastatic renal cell carcinoma. J Neurosurg Spine 2016;25(6):766–74.

75. Kumar R, Nater A, Hashmi A, et al. The era of stereotactic body radiotherapy for spinal metastases and the multidisciplinary management of complex cases. Neurooncol Pract 2015;3(1):48–58.

76. Sohn S, Chung CK, Sohn MJ, et al. Stereotactic radiosurgery compared with external radiation therapy as a primary treatment in spine metastasis from renal cell carcinoma: a multicenter, matched-pair study. J Neurooncol 2014;119(1):121–8.

77. Ganju RG, TenNapel M, Mahan N, et al. The efficacy of conventionally fractionated radiation in the management of osseous metastases from metastatic renal cell carcinoma. J Oncol 2018;2018:6384253.

78. Amini A, Altoos B, Bourlon MT, et al. Local control rates of metastatic renal cell carcinoma (RCC) to the bone using stereotactic body radiation therapy: Is RCC truly radioresistant? Pract Radiat Oncol 2015;5(6):e589–96.

79. DiBiase SJ, Valicenti RK, Schultz D, et al. Palliative irradiation for focally symptomatic metastatic renal cell carcinoma: support for dose escalation based on a biological model. J Urol 1997;158(3 Pt 1): 746–9.

80. Wersall PJ, Blomgren H, Lax I, et al. Extracranial stereotactic radiotherapy for primary and metastatic renal cell carcinoma. Radiother Oncol 2005;77(1): 88–95.

81. Ranck MC, Golden DW, Corbin KS, et al. Stereotactic body radiotherapy for the treatment of oligometastatic renal cell carcinoma. Am J Clin Oncol 2013; 36(6):589–95.

82. Zaorsky NG, Lehrer EJ, Kothari G, et al. Stereotactic ablative radiation therapy for oligometastatic renal cell carcinoma (SABR ORCA): a meta-analysis of 28 studies. Eur Urol Oncol 2019;2(5):515–23.

83. Singh AK, Winslow TB, Kermany MH, et al. A pilot study of stereotactic body radiation therapy combined with cytoreductive nephrectomy for metastatic renal cell carcinoma. Clin Cancer Res 2017;23(17): 5055–65.

84. Zhang Y, Schoenhals J, Christie A, et al. Stereotactic ablative radiation therapy (SAbR) used to defer systemic therapy in oligometastatic renal cell cancer. Int J Radiat Oncol Biol Phys 2019;105(2):367–75.

85. LaPlant Q, Deselm C, Lockney NA, et al. Potential abscopal response to dual checkpoint blockade in RCC after reirradiation using dose-painting SBRT. Pract Radiat Oncol 2017;7(6):396–9.

86. Van de Walle M, Demol J, Staelens L, et al. Abscopal effect in metastatic renal cell carcinoma. Acta Clin Belg 2017;72(4):245–9.

87. Solanki AA, Bossi A, Efstathiou JA, et al. Combining immunotherapy with radiotherapy for the treatment of genitourinary malignancies. Eur Urol Oncol 2019;2(1):79–87.

88. Schöggl A, Kitz K, Ertl A, et al. Gamma-knife radiosurgery for brain metastases of renal cell carcinoma: results in 23 patients. Acta Neurochir (Wien) 1998; 140(6):549–55.

89. Kim WH, Kim DG, Han JH, et al. Early significant tumor volume reduction after radiosurgery in brain metastases from renal cell carcinoma results in long-term survival. Int J Radiat Oncol Biol Phys 2012;82(5):1749–55.

90. Stenman M, Sinclair G, Paavola P, et al. Overall survival after stereotactic radiotherapy or surgical metastasectomy in oligometastatic renal cell carcinoma patients treated at two Swedish centres 2005-2014. Radiother Oncol 2018;127(3):501–6.

91. Franzese C, Franceschini D, Di Brina L, et al. Role of stereotactic body radiation therapy for the management of oligometastatic renal cell carcinoma. J Urol 2019;201(1):70–6.

Moving?

Make sure your subscription moves with you!

To notify us of your new address, find your **Clinics Account Number** (located on your mailing label above your name), and contact customer service at:

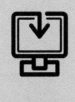

Email: journalscustomerservice-usa@elsevier.com

800-654-2452 (subscribers in the U.S. & Canada)
314-447-8871 (subscribers outside of the U.S. & Canada)

Fax number: 314-447-8029

Elsevier Health Sciences Division
Subscription Customer Service
3251 Riverport Lane
Maryland Heights, MO 63043

*To ensure uninterrupted delivery of your subscription, please notify us at least 4 weeks in advance of move.

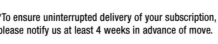
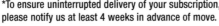

Printed and bound by CPI Group (UK) Ltd, Croydon, CR0 4YY

03/10/2024

01040306-0016